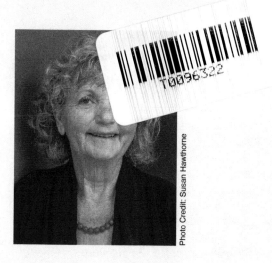

Dr Renate Klein is a long-term women's health researcher and has written extensively on reproductive technologies and feminist theory over the last 30 years. A biologist and social scientist, she was Associate Professor in Women's Studies at Deakin University in Melbourne. She is a co-founder of FINRRAGE (Feminist International Network of Resistance to Reproductive and Genetic Engineering) and an original signatory to Stop Surrogacy Now.

Other books by Renate Klein

RU 486: Misconceptions, Myths and Morals
(2013/1991, with Janice G Raymond and Lynette J Dumble)

Horse Dreams: The Meaning of Horses in Women's Lives
(2004, co-edited with Jan Fook and Susan Hawthorne)

Cat Tales: The Meaning of Cats in Women's Lives
(2003, co-edited with Jan Fook and Susan Hawthorne)

A Girl's Best Friend: The Meaning of Dogs in Women's Lives
(2001, co-edited with Jan Fook)

CyberFeminism: Connectivity, Critique and Creativity
(1999, co-edited with Susan Hawthorne)

Radically Speaking: Feminism Reclaimed
(1996, co-edited with Diane Bell)

Australia for Women: Travel and Culture
(1994, co-edited with Susan Hawthorne)

The Ultimate Colonisation: Reproductive and Genetic Engineering
(1992)

Angels of Power and Other Reproductive Creations
(1991, co-edited with Susan Hawthorne)

Radical Voices: A Decade of Resistance from Women's Studies International Forum (1989, co-edited with Deborah L Steinberg)

Infertility: Women Speak Out about Their Experiences with Reproductive Medicine (1989, editor)

The Exploitation of a Desire: Women's Experiences with in Vitro Fertilisation (1989)

Man-made Women: How New Reproductive Technologies Affect Women
(1985/1987, co-authored with Gena Corea *et al.*)

Test-Tube Women: What Future for Motherhood?
(1984, co-edited with Rita Arditti and Shelley Minden)

Theories of Women's Studies
(1983, co-edited with Gloria Bowles)

Feministische Wissenschaft und Frauenstudium
(1982, co-edited with Sigrid Metz-Göckel and Maresi Nerad)

Surrogacy

A Human Rights Violation

Renate Klein

First published by Spinifex Press, Australia, 2017 - Reprinted 2017

Spinifex Press Pty Ltd
PO Box 5270, North Geelong, Victoria 3215
PO Box 105, Mission Beach, Queensland 4852
Australia

women@spinifexpress.com.au
www.spinifexpress.com.au

Cover image by Estelle Disch
Cover design by Deb Snibson, MAPG
Edited by Pauline Hopkins and Susan Hawthorne
Indexed by Karen Gillen
Typeset in Australia by Blue Wren Books
Typeset in Utopia
Printed by McPherson's Printing Group

National Library of Australia Cataloguing-in-Publication
Klein, Renate, author.
Surrogacy : a human rights violation / Renate Klein.

ISBN: 9781925581034 (paperback)
ISBN: 9781925581041 (ebook : pdf)
ISBN: 9781925581065 (ebook : epub)
ISBN: 9781925581058 (ebook : Kindle)

Series: Spinifex shorts.
Includes bibliographical references and index.
Human reproductive technology.
Surrogate motherhood–Moral and ethical aspects.
Human rights.

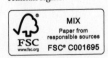

It is a fundamental premise of international law that the rights of human beings must be based on human dignity.

—Gena Corea, 1989, p. 263

Contents

Acknowledgements

I have been working as a critic of reproductive technologies and genetic engineering including surrogacy for a long time: since the beginning of the 1980s. It is thus quite impossible to mention all my friends and colleagues with whom I have laughed and cried and demonstrated at rallies and talked at conferences over more than 30 years. And written papers and books with, edited journals, exchanged many letters (especially before emails), but also shared our vision for a better and fairer world in which patriarchal violence both in the sexual exploitation – and reproductive – industries would abate. I can't name and thank you all, but will mention a few: my co-founding members of FINRRAGE (Feminist International Network of Resistance to Reproductive and Genetic Engineering) and dear friends, Janice Raymond, Robyn Rowland, Farida Akhter, Jalna Hanmer and Maria Mies, my inspirations Gena Corea and Rita Arditti: my life would have been so much emptier without your presence that continues to this day. And much less happy, because in spite of our heartbreaking topic and doggedly hard work, we shared many good times and hearty laughs. Other longtime FINRRAGE members and friends who have shared and supported my journey include Lariane Fonseca, Melinda Tankard Reist, Annette Burfoot, Erika Feyerabend, Kathy Munro,

Delanie Woodlock, Laurel Guymer, Ana Regina Gomes Dos Reis, Mary Sullivan, Selena Ewing, Simone Watson, Helen Pringle, Isla MacGregor and Coleen Clare.

The reproductive exploitation of women became front-page news again in the first decade of the 21st century when cloning was hailed as the newest grail of the scientific quest to save us from all imperfection. This demanded easy access to thousands of women's egg cells for embryonic stem cell research. In 2006, I joined with old and new friends in a sister organisation to FINRRAGE, Hands Off Our Ovaries. When the hype of this miracle technology began to fade (as we had predicted it would), cross-border surrogacy began to rear its ugly head: bigger than ever again. So in 2015, I again joined with old and new friends to oppose this latest phase of ruthless exploitation of vulnerable women and their children in the new activist campaign Stop Surrogacy Now. Members are everywhere in the world and again too numerous to list and thank, but let me just highlight a few women here. Above all tremendous credit goes to Jennifer Lahl without whose vision and boundless energy Stop Surrogacy Now would not have gotten off the ground and expanded to more than 8000 supporters by July 2017. But I also want to thank Kajsa Ekis Ekman, Kathy Sloan, Penny Mackieson, Jo Fraser, Julie Bindel and yet again Janice Raymond and Melinda Tankard Reist for their ongoing sterling work. We may not be able to finish off the dirty global surrogacy business exploiting vulnerable people any time soon, but hopefully we can shine some public light on their ruthless operations and also hold a mirror to the faces of those fence-sitting, wishy-washy harms minimisation liberals who could join with us and make our work truly move mountains!

A special thank you goes to Stevie de Saille who put hard work, but also her heart and soul into her PhD on FINRRAGE and then into her forthcoming book *Knowledge as Resistance: The Feminist International Network of Resistance to Reproductive and Genetic Engineering* (2018). When Stevie came to Australia on a fellowship in 2010, Robyn Rowland and I spent many happy hours in memory-land with her. We are grateful and excited about your book. Thank you Stevie!

This small book – one of the Spinifex 'Shorts' – took longer to write than it should have, not only because of other ongoing work commitments, but also because of the tragic death within 24 hours of our beloved Dingo-Dog Freya in the prime of her life in January 2016. This unexpected tragedy sent both me and my partner into a months' long spiral of deepest sorrow and grief, only helped by co-dog lovers' support: thank you to Vicky Black, Debbie Orenshaw, Estelle Disch and Nelly Hearn who often cried with us for our and their own dogs' loss. And thank you to Betty McLellan who kept me going on Words with Friends (although you win too often), and to Doris Hermanns who supported me with a significant amount of Lindt pralinés in Berlin and kept (somewhat irritatingly) asking "have you finished it yet?" Finally Doris, I can say "yes, I have."

I also thank everyone at Spinifex Press who kept believing that one day there would be a final manuscript: Susan Hawthorne, Pauline Hopkins, Helen Lobato and Maralann Damiano. I am incredibly grateful to Pauline for digging up obscure TV and other media references, and to Susan and Pauline for overall greatly improving the quality of this short 'fat' book. Delanie Woodlock also contributed some initial editing, thank you to all. Any remaining 'Swissisms' and shortcomings are of course my own responsibility.

And finally, how do I thank Susan Hawthorne, my partner of 30 years, and co-publisher of Spinifex Press for 25 years, for her incredible patience with hearing me rage about reproductive technologies and surrogacy for ... yes, 30 years. It takes a very special love and friendship to keep reading drafts, fume with me about the latest iterations of woman-hating technologies, and cook beautiful meals whilst at the same time finishing her own inspirational novel *Dark Matters*. There can never be enough 'thank yous' to Susan who remains my best friend, true love, co-mourner of Freya and River, and hopefully, one day, co-companion of a new dog friend.

Mission Beach, July 2017

A word on language: Since I don't agree that 'surrogate' mother is an appropriate term to describe a woman who grows a baby in her womb for nine months, and argue that there is nothing 'surrogate' about this process, in this book, I always place the term in quotation marks. I do the same with egg 'donor', as donation (of sperm or blood for instance) is totally different from the invasive and dangerous procedures of producing high numbers of ripe egg cells in an ovary and then 'harvesting' them. This makes for somewhat cumbersome reading and I apologise. But it can't be helped. Sometimes I use the term egg provider which I don't like either, but find preferable to 'donor'. I also put inverted commas around words or expressions that I don't like (or want to make a sarcastic comment about). As there are many in a discussion of surrogacy, this book is littered with them. Again my apologies, but dear reader, it is important to hear what the mainstream media and literature won't tell you. I use Commonwealth English throughout the text but leave quotations in US English (and yes that's done on purpose, hello to my readers in the USA and Canada!).

Introduction

The 21st century is witnessing a rapid expansion of the surrogacy industry, both commercial and so-called altruistic. Although surrogacy has been a profitable and largely unregulated trade in women and their babies since the 1980s in the USA and soon after in India, the last decade has seen commercial surrogacy, including egg 'donation', boom in many poor countries of Eastern Europe and Asia. When a disaster occurs – such as the sad case in 2014 of Down syndrome Baby Gammy left behind in Thailand by his Australian commissioning sex-offender father and his wife (see p. 39), or the Indian government excluding gay couples from surrogacy in 2013, and all foreign couples in 2015,[1] the industry responds by shifting to new countries such as Nepal, Malaysia, and Cambodia. And when yet another government prohibits surrogacy for foreigners (Nepal and the Mexican province of Tabasco in 2015), or another

---

1   'India bans gay foreign couples from surrogacy' (18 January 2013); <http://www.telegraph.co.uk/news/worldnews/asia/india/9811222/India-bans-gay-foreign-couples-from-surrogacy.html>; 'Foreign Couples in Limbo After India Restricts Surrogacy Services' (16 November 2015); <https://www.wsj.com/articles/foreign-couples-in-limbo-after-india-restricts-surrogacy-services-1447698601>

scandal breaks – as happened in Cambodia in 2016[2] – yet another location opens, such as Laos. And Ukraine, with its new high-tech IVF centers, is vying for customers in enticing videos.

Surrogacy is heavily promoted by the stagnating IVF industry which seeks new markets, as well as by gay men who believe they have a 'right' to their own children and 'family foundation'. Pro-surrogacy lobby groups in rich countries such as Australia and Western Europe (which allow only 'altruistic' surrogacy or no surrogacy at all) push for the shift to commercial surrogacy. Their capitalist neoliberal argument is that a well-regulated fertility industry would avoid the exploitative practices of poor countries. Indeed, considerable efforts are going into a regulatory scheme that would see surrogacy become an acceptable practice in affluent countries spearheaded by neo-liberal lawyers, academics, counsellors and liberal feminists. Their aims include the creation of a global Hague Convention on surrogacy – thereby legally cementing the commodification of women, and production of children, in surrogacy as 'work' under the guise of transnational labour laws.[3]

Central to the project of (international) surrogacy is the ideology that legalised commercial surrogacy is a legitimate means to providing infertile couples and gay men with children who share all, or part of, their genes. Women, without whose

---

2   'Australian nurse Tammy Davis-Charles arrested in Cambodian surrogacy crackdown' (20 November 2016); <http://www.smh.com.au/world/australian-nurse-tammy-charles-caught-up-in-cambodian-surrogacy-crackdown-20161120-gstd23.html>

3   <http://www.abc.net.au/news/2014-08-21/van-whichelen-what-chance-for-international-surrogacy-laws/5683746>

bodies this project is not possible – not yet at least as the artificial womb has still not been perfected (see Conclusion, pp. 162–167) – are reduced to incubators, to ovens, to suitcases. And the product child is a tradable commodity who of course has never consented to being a 'take-away baby': removed from their birth mother and given to strangers aka 'intended parents'. Still, those in favour of this practice of reproductive slavery believe it can be regulated and made into 'Fair Trade International Surrogacy' (Humbyrd, 2009; Pande 2017) and 'Responsible Surrogacy'.[4]

The comparison with the sex trade is obvious: well-regulated sex (or fertility) industries, according to their promoters, create happy hookers (happy surrogates) and happy sex buyers (happy baby buyers). Pimps and brothel owners equal IVF clinics, surrogacy lawyers/brokers, pro-surrogacy advocacy groups, as well as surrogacy/egg 'donor' agencies. The difference is that apart from deeply harming women in both industries, the end 'product' in prostitution is a 'faked girlfriend experience', whereas in surrogacy it is the creation of new human beings: children.

It is obvious from these opening lines that I thoroughly disagree with the theory and practice of surrogacy, both as a regulated capitalist enterprise and as a form of uncompensated 'altruistic love'. Instead I believe it is a violation of the human rights of the egg 'donor', the birth mother and the resulting child(ren).

---

4   The website for Responsible Surrogacy reveals that it simply offers to regulate the practice, see Chapter 5 for a critique of regulation; <http://www.r-surrogacy.org/en/>

In the following pages, I will detail my objections to surrogacy, firstly, by asking the question "what is surrogacy?" Next, I examine the short- and long-term harms done to the so-called surrogates, egg providers and the female partner in a heterosexual commissioning couple and briefly address the (tedious) question of whether this constitutes 'choice'. Then I will look at the rights of children and compare surrogacy to (forced) adoption practices. Other crucial questions are: "can surrogacy be ethical?," "would it be ethical if we called it 'work'?" and, "is regulation the answer?" Next, I will outline past and current forms of resistance and in the Conclusion look at the 'Background' of reproductive technologies and inquire how far we have come with developments of an artificial womb. Finally I make my plea for this dehumanising industry to be stopped and not gain further traction in patriarchal mainstream society.

Chapter 1
What is surrogacy?

Pared down to cold hard facts, surrogacy is the commissioning/ buying/renting of a woman into whose womb an embryo is inserted and who thus becomes a 'breeder' for a third party.

In a 'traditional' surrogacy, the 'surrogate' is inseminated with the sperm from the husband/partner of the commissioning heterosexual couple. The sperm fuses with her own egg cell(s) and creates an embryo which then, if successful, implants itself in her womb.

If the partner/wife is infertile, an egg 'donor' will provide egg cells that are fertilised in the laboratory with the husband's/ partner's sperm. This is called 'gestational surrogacy'. In the case of two gay men who can only ever provide sperm, an egg donor is always necessary.

'Traditional' surrogacy is rarely done any more because, with this method, the birth mother's genes form half of the child's genetic heritage, apparently making her more prone to resist relinquishing her baby.

But also, if 'gestational' surrogacy which always needs in vitro-fertilisation (IVF) is used, this is a much better source of income for fertility clinics as they get new clients: the egg 'donors' and the so-called surrogate mothers. Moreover, the embryo created from the donor eggs and buyer(s)' sperm can be subjected to prenatal genetic diagnosis (PGD) before it is inserted in the rented woman's body. In this way, more money can be made from multiple screening tests for abnormalities and sex selection (where allowed) which is nothing short of eugenics in action. Because IVF pregnancies continue to have a high *failure* rate – still close to 80% according to UK IVF Pioneer Lord Winston[5] – surplus embryos can be frozen and more surrogacy cycles can be sold.

The parties involved in these transactions include a fertility clinic with IVF doctors, a surrogacy law firm (in the US often a surrogacy broker), a surrogacy agency with a register of available 'surrogates', and an egg 'donor' agency with suitable young and good looking women on their website. And there are third-party surrogacy facilitators who oversee transnational egg and embryo transfers, and, in some cases, counsellors. New business opportunities are aplenty with enterprises such as 'Eggspecting', 'Complete Surrogacy Solutions', 'Surrogacy Beyond Borders', 'Family Inceptions International' and many more. Importantly

---

5   IVF 'pioneers' Robert Winston and Robert Edwards now warn that the hormonal drugs used in 'assisted reproduction' are producing '... chromosomal damage in at least half, if not 70%, of eggs (Winston quoted in Marsh, 2006). This is an astounding admission after decades of defending the use of an ever-increasing range of fertility drugs (and denouncing radical feminist research that found such evidence already in the 1980s, e.g. Klein/Rowland, 1988). During his 2007 visit to Australia, Robert Winston also stated on the *7:30 Report* on ABC Television (12 July 2007) that the success rate from IVF was 15 to 20%: at long last a realistic assessment that, together with the worrying news about health problems in children born from IVF, hopefully will make people think twice before embarking on IVF or, indeed, surrogacy.

also, there are pro-surrogacy advocacy groups such as 'Families Through Surrogacy' in Australia who organise yearly (inter-) national conferences, offer advice on transnational surrogacy, and 'altruistic' surrogacy at home, put prospective parents in touch with egg 'donors' and women willing to act as 'surrogates'. 'Grooming' is another term to describe these activities.

Then there is the so-called surrogate, a misnomer as this is a woman who will grow the baby for nine months from her own body and give birth to it. In commercial surrogacy, this birth mother is always from a lower socio-economic class and often also from a different 'lower-ranked' ethnicity than the commissioning couple. Race and class issues abound: we are yet to see a (white-skinned) CEO who carries a baby for her (brown-skinned) cleaner. The surrogacy/egg 'donation' transactions are between well-off people and poor(er) women. Going to countries such as India, Cambodia or Ukraine because of much lower prices means that the 'surrogates' are inevitably poor women with little education, often kept in prison-like camps for the duration of their pregnancy and often 'pimped' by their husbands who have come to see surrogacy as a lucrative income-generating scheme (Sangari, 2015, p. 120).

In 'altruistic' surrogacy in which no money is supposed to change hands (except quite considerable payments for 'expenses'), it is often fertile family members such as sisters, cousins or aunts who are so moved by the plight of their infertile relatives – or gay family members – that they offer their bodies (and souls) for this self-sacrificing 'service'. Changing their mind about the growing baby is next to impossible as that would involve being ostracised from their families. When it is non-family members who become altruistic 'surrogates', they dissociate from the child growing in their bodies: "not my baby but my passenger, he was just sitting on my bus for a while."[6]

After nine months, the resulting baby is removed, usually by Caesarean section, and handed over to the 'commissioning parents' who pay the final instalment for their product(s), often twins. Child buying or child trafficking is a suitable term for such transactions. The connection between birth mother and the new parents is either non-existent from the day of birth, or, mostly, short-lived. The child(ren) only rarely will have a connection to the woman who grew them from her own flesh, bones and blood and retains some of her baby's cells for decades (Dawe, Tan, and Xiao, 2007).

The child buyers put their names on the birth certificate[7] and name themselves the baby's 'parents', rationalising that it is the sperm donor's genes who are in this child, hence it is his and has no connection to its birth mother. Strangely, in this tale of alleged gene superiority that bestows child ownership, the genes of the egg provider, if there was one, are routinely 'forgotten' –

---

6   A statement made by Australian 'altruistic' surrogate Renee Gollard in 2015 on a panel discussion after the play e-Baby by Jane Cafarella on 8 March, 2015 in Melbourne. See also <http://www.abc.net.au/radionational/programs/drawingroom/e-baby/6273604>

7   This may take place immediately after birth, or, as in the state of Victoria in Australia, the commissioning parents have to first apply through the courts for a substitute parentage order. See <https://www.bdm.vic.gov.au/births/donor-conceived-births/surrogacy> and <https://www.varta.org.au/information-support/surrogacy/commissioning-parents/surrogacy-australia/legal-side-surrogacy>

another woman who is crucial to the process of gestation – but does not matter. That the children might want to know at some point who gave them half of their genes, appears to be of no concern.

Naturally, this version of surrogacy has a fairy tale ending: The commissioning parents are besotted with their child(ren) and love them to bits. They dress them in pink or blue designer clothes and enrol them in programs for gifted pre-schoolers. The children turn out super intelligent and well behaved. They neither ask about, nor miss, the two women who contributed to their existence – the birth mother and the woman who provided the egg cell – and grow into happy, well adjusted, high achieving, teenagers and adults.

These 'bare facts' of surrogacy of course leave out the traumas that can arise during the 'manufacturing process': the quality of the sperm or the donor's egg cells are inferior; the embryo transfer fails; the developing embryo is 'imperfect' and needs to be aborted; the 'surrogate' refuses an abortion and a 'defect' baby is born (as happened in the Baby Gammy case); the 'surrogate' mother falls ill, miscarries or dies; the commissioning couple divorces, or one partner dies; the 'surrogate' mother changes her mind during pregnancy and wants to keep the child. Or the couple did not do their homework and are now stranded in a far away country with 'their' baby for whom their home country is not issuing a visa – as has happened to citizens from Switzerland, France, Germany and Norway.[8]

---

8   <http://www.swissinfo.ch/eng/surrogate-law_a-child-is-not-a-commodity--says-top-swiss-court/41575816>

Of course, those who support surrogacy and believe that someone's individualistic *desire* for a child equals the *need* for – and gives them the *right* to – a child, whatever the price, and whoever gets left behind on this journey, will vehemently disagree with my description of surrogacy so far. For them, surrogacy is a precious act of wonder and kindness.

Similarly, those in the liberal harms-reduction camp will find my words harsh: surely these practices can be regulated and exploitation can be minimised. They will accuse me of unkindness: I must be a heartless person who has no understanding of the profound grief and despair infertility can cause, or in the case of two men, their inability to give birth to a child themselves.

To them I reply that as a matter of fact I do understand only too well. My research into Australian women's experiences with IVF in the 1980s (Klein 1989a) as well as editing major feminist anthologies on new reproductive technologies (Arditti, Duelli Klein and Minden, 1984; Klein 1989b) led me to experience many instances in my interviews with women undergoing IVF where their desperation about wanting a child was heartbreaking. Because IVF was (and is) traumatic and the failure rates were (and are) enormous (then 90%, today 70% to 80% depending on age and honest reporting by the clinics), for many women it was still possible to stop the brutal IVF journey and find other ways of having children in their lives. They had the support of much of their community who helped them through this sad period in their lives. Alas this changed in the 21st century: with egg 'donation' and surrogacy the new 'products' on the IVF clinics' supermarket shelves, and regularly featured glowingly in women's magazines when yet another celebrity had a 'surrogate' child. Women who are in their 40s and have gone through IVF ten to fifteen times (and are deep in financial debt already) are not allowed to stop. Another woman will now 'gift' them an egg cell, and a second woman will carry 'her' baby (and the fee paying – as well as the anxiety – will continue).

Their ultimate 'uselessness' as a 'proper' woman confirmed by their family as well as society at large, they must now welcome this arrangement, be thankful to the IVF clinic for their miracle work – and hide their pain. And of course then be the perfect and joyful mother to another woman's child – if there is one. Or repeat the process until a baby is born.

In addition to accusing any critic of surrogacy of callousness, without fail there is a strident chorus of pro-surrogacy voices invoking 'choice', 'consent' and 'a woman's right to her body', thus invariably accusing critics of presenting women as helpless victims: 'Surrogates' consent to what they do. Egg 'donors' know which procedures await them (and are handsomely paid). These women do it because they want to be life-givers, and their customers love them for it – calling them heroes and angels – and profoundly thanking them for their gift. And, in the rare cases when dodgy players might be involved, *regulation* is the best way to ensure problems are prevented before they occur (see Chapter 5 for details on regulation).

I disagree with these assessments. In the next section, I will examine the harms suffered by the women involved in surrogacy, and briefly discuss questions of 'choice', 'consent' and 'self-determination'.

Chapter 2
Short- and long-term harms of surrogacy

In surrogacy, three women are harmed: the 'surrogate' mother, the egg provider and the female partner in a heterosexual commissioning couple.[9]

The part of the process to achieve a pregnancy is the most invasive in terms of daily drug injections necessary to 'ready' the womb and the endocrine system of the 'surrogate' mother for the embryo insertion. For the egg provider (who is a third party, or the female partner), this phase involves putting her first into chemical menopause and then dousing her with fertility drugs for superovulation: the production of dozens of good healthy egg cells that can be extracted and then fertilised by the buyer's sperm to create embryos.

Daily painful injections, headaches, nausea, cramping, becoming bloated, feeling sick, dizzy and emotional and putting on weight are just some of the unavoidable adverse effects. Ovarian hyperstimulation syndrome (OHSS) can be

---

9   Of course other family members can also be harmed, e.g. the 'surrogate' mother's partner, her children; the commissioning parents' families who may fundamentally disagree with surrogacy and/or put blame on their daughter/daughter-in-law or son/son-in-law for being unable to 'naturally' produce a child.

life threatening and has resulted in serious injury such as pulmonary complications (when the lungs fill with fluid which needs to be extracted), stroke, and death. Equally worrying are the largely unknown long-term adverse effects of the drugs. Many of them, such as Lupron (leuprolide acetate), are used 'off-label', which means that they were never registered for use in IVF/egg 'donation' and as a consequence, no research was conducted to find out about any short- or long-term adverse effects when used in women. (In the USA the FDA registered Lupron as treatment for prostate cancer.[10]) It is a breathtaking and world-wide scandal that no country has ever mandated its IVF clinics to undertake short- and long-term follow-up of the health of women undergoing IVF, and compare ill health with the drugs that were used in individual treatments.

This is good news for pharmaceutical companies because such are the variations in drugs used in IVF since the early 1980s that, even if comprehensive studies were finally retrospectively undertaken, it will be impossible to link certain long-term adverse effects such as ovarian, uterine and breast cancer with

---

10 The website <www.lupronvictimshub/lawsuits.html> lists the lawsuits against the manufacturer of Lupron. The site is administered by former psychiatric nurse Lynne Millican who has written extensively about her own adverse reactions to the drug. She reports that the first plaintiff to make it to trial in the USA was Karin Klein in 2011; <https://impactethics. ca/2014/05/02/hidden-clinical-trial-data-about-lupron/> Lupron is also used as a puberty blocker in 'tall girls' and in the increasing number of so-called transgender children. The drug has serious adverse effects on bone health, and young women in their twenties have reported serious degenerate disc disease and bone thinning. It is a big problem that needs urgent attention (see Jewett, 2 February 2017).

specific drugs. At best what might be established is that women who underwent IVF end up with higher rates of these cancers, but not which drug(s) caused them. Or else it is the women themselves who are blamed for the higher cancer rates.

This is what happened in October 2015 when a relatively large study that included 250,000 IVF users in the UK between 1991 and 2010 concluded that these women had a one-third greater chance of developing ovarian cancer.[11] Immediately women were reassured that firstly, these numbers weren't very large, and secondly, it was not possible to prove 'cause and effect' of whether any of the IVF drugs were responsible for the increased number of ovarian cancers. Rather, the researchers suggested it was likely that infertility or 'childlessness' itself might be the cause(s) of the higher cancer rates.

End of story, panic averted, back to IVF business as usual which of course includes 'surrogate' mothers and especially egg 'providers' who often undergo the 'eggsploitation' procedure many times.[12] 'Eggsploitation' is the name of a powerful documentary produced by the US Center for Bioethics and Culture (2010–2013). Through interviews with US women who

---

11 The lead researcher for the study was Alastair Sutcliffe from University College London. The article appeared on <http://www.fertstert.org/article/S0015-0282(15)00614-7/fulltext>

12 *Confessions of a Serial Egg Donor* (2004) by Julia Derek makes for insightful but disturbing reading. A blond and beautiful Swedish student who had arrived in the USA found it hard to pay for her college tuition, Derek turned to 'donating' eggs. Despite getting very sick and being hospitalised for life-threatening illness, she had eggs extracted twelve times – until her body finally shut down. Her book exposes the lure of money and the callousness of egg brokers who put profit before the health of egg 'donors'.

had 'donated' their eggs as well as with health practitioners, the documentary shows the serious dangers inherent in the process.[13]

This might be a good moment to address the point so much laboured by neoliberals (feminists included), pro-surrogacy advocacy groups, brokers, IVF clinics, and regurgitated by the mainstream media, namely that it is a woman's 'choice' and 'self-determination' to become a 'surrogate' or egg 'donor', and that 'surrogates' have made their 'free choice' with 'informed consent.'

'Choice' is a word I would be happy to ban (had I the power). I suggest it should only be used to differentiate between two *good* things such as "Do you want a piece of chocolate cake or the lemon tart?" Used only in this way, we would immediately get rid of it in difficult situations where *both* outcomes are excruciating. To 'choose' to stay in prostitution when you have become heavily addicted to cocaine, desperately need money, are homeless and have not a soul to turn to for support, is not a 'choice': it is a most difficult (and unfortunate) decision. Likewise, to 'choose' to exploit a woman as a 'surrogate' when your family including your husband blames you for being infertile and treats you like an outcast, is not a 'choice': it is a most difficult (and unfortunate) decision.

---

13 In 2015, the Center for Bioethics and Culture also produced a follow up documentary 'Maggie's story' that tells the sad story of Maggie who ended up with advanced breast cancer after more than ten egg extractions. Another excellent documentary on the subject of surrogacy is called 'Breeders: A Subclass of Women?' (2014), see <http://breeders.cbc-network.org>

The reverse situation is to 'choose' to become a 'surrogate' or an egg 'donor' because your husband pushes you when your yearly salary in an Indian garment factory is a fraction of what you can earn as a 'womb mother' in nine months. Or when a man's salary from the US army gets a nice lift when his wife becomes an 'army surrogate' – entirely voluntarily, of course. Again, whatever the outcome, these are not 'choices' but (often difficult) *decisions*.

We should never blame women for decisions they make at particular times in their lives. But we should stop calling them 'choices' *without taking into account the social context within which women make decisions*. These decisions often lead to practices that harm them greatly (but without fail, fill the coffers of the greedy sexual exploitation and reproduction industries).[14]

---

14 When new reproductive technologies including surrogacy were initially put under feminist scrutiny in the 1980s, there was a plethora of writings on the question of 'choice' and informed consent. For excellent books on this topic see Robyn Rowland's *Living Laboratories* from Australia (1992) and Janice Raymond's *Women as Wombs* from the USA (1993/1995). In German-speaking countries it was a groundbreaking speech by feminist sociologist Maria Mies in 1988 on self-determination ('Selbstbestimmung – Das Ende einer Utopie?'; 'Self-determination – The End of an Utopia?', in Bradish *et al.*, 1988). In her talk, delivered to an electrified audience of over 2000 women opposed to gene and reproductive technologies in Frankfurt (and later expanded), Mies pointed out the nonsense of continuing to use the terms 'self-determination' or 'choice' as our feminist battle cry (a leftover from women's demand for abortion rights). As she pointed out, gene and reproductive technologies have reduced our bodies to fragmented 'objects' that are now being controlled by outsiders: the state, IVF clinics, surrogacy brokers and Big Pharma. No longer 'Self-determination', it is now 'Other-determination'. And in the so-called third world, Mies points out, 'self-determination' for women has been reduced to 'choosing' between

Most importantly, we have to robustly reject the accusations by pro-surrogacy advocates when they say that abolitionists disparage women with our opposition. As US ethicist Janice Raymond put it succinctly (1993/1995, p. x, my emphasis):

> Choice so dominates the discussion that when critics of technological reproduction denounce the ways in which women are abused by these procedures, we are accused of making women into victims and, supposedly, of denying that women are capable of choice. *To expose the victimization of women is to be blamed for creating women as victims.*

Indeed this was precisely what played out in Australia in 2006/2007 when a Commonwealth Bill considered an Amendment allowing embryonic stem cell research which necessitates women to 'donate' egg cells.

Feminist groups including FINRRAGE (Australia) and Hands Off Our Ovaries[15] opposed the Amendment on the grounds that female relatives of severely ill or injured people will be under pressure to 'do the right thing' and 'donate' egg cells when

---

which pills – the green ones or the pink ones – will limit their fertility and harm them.

15 The inspiring international Hands Off Our Ovaries Campaign (HOOO) was started in 2006 by a group of three pro-choice and two pro-life feminists from the UK, Canada and the USA, and supported by thousands of signatories around the world. Unfortunately, after a few years of great advocacy work it dwindled away when the US pro-choice liberal feminist members gave in to pressure from within their own ranks that an alliance with pro-life feminists – entirely focused on women, not embryos I must point out – was too risky: a most regrettable decision that says a lot about the rigidity of (US) liberal feminists. In many ways HOOO was the precursor of Stop Surrogacy Now, established in 2015 (see Chapter 6, pp. 145–153).

embryonic cloning advocates wax lyrical about the life-saving treatments they will be able to develop for debilitating incurable degenerative motor neurone disease or spinal cord injuries. We pointed out that information about egg 'donation' lacked details about short- and long-term risks (and the fact that long-term research was sorely lacking), so potential egg 'donors' would be unable to provide proper 'informed consent' and exercise 'choice'.

Swiftly, we were accused by the then most vocal pro-choice abortion activist, Leslie Cannold, of being 'sexist' and infantilising and patronising women. She argued that no one should have the right "... to stop me or any other women, making my own risk-benefit calculation, and my own choice" (Cannold, 2006).

So the 'rhetoric of choice' (Klein, 2006) was used big time by advocates of the Amendment to divert attention away from having a much-needed public discussion of the risks of egg 'donation'. It was easier to condemn feminists and wrongly accuse us of saying that women "... lack the *capacity* to give informed consent to egg donation" (Cannold, 2006, my emphasis).[16] Of course, it is not women who lack the 'capacity'; the point is that they are not given the facts (or the facts do not exist).

---

16 The Prohibition of Human Cloning and the Regulation of Human Embryo Research Amendment Bill 2006 (*Commonwealth of Australia,* 2006) was eventually passed with just one vote by a member of parliament who voted in favour of research safeguards for animals rather than women. However, Leslie Cannold had done herself no favours by comparing the procedures involved in egg 'donation' with donating blood, which she said, "... – like all medical procedures – carries risks" (Cannold 2006).

Returning to the specifics of egg 'donation', a perusal of a dozen IVF websites is enough to see that the possibility of serious adverse effects is not mentioned. As one woman put it succinctly in 'Eggsploitation': "They don't fill you in on the health risks." Even the rare mention that there might be some 'unlikely' long-term problems such as an increased number of cancers, is still incorrect. What ought to be said to all women considering 'donating' eggs or going through IVF is that in fact the studies have not been done, the research is not there: *no one knows what the health risks are!*[17]

Eggsploitation is defined succinctly in the documentary:

To plunder, pillage, rob, despoil, fleece, and strip ruthlessly a young woman of her eggs, by means of fraud, coercion or deception, to be used selfishly for another's gain, with a total lack of regard for the well being of the donor.

Of course, the egg 'donation' story does not end with the drugs. Egg harvesting which takes place under anaesthesia with a needle inserted through the vagina, then piercing the ovaries and sucking ripe egg follicles out, can lead to the loss of an ovary when the puncture wounds become infected, or blood vessels

---

17 This is precisely what Jennifer Schneider and colleagues published in *Reproductive BioMedicine Online* in 2017. While reviewing the literature on adverse effects after egg provision for higher rates of breast cancer, they found a host of contradictory studies: some finding higher rates of breast (and ovarian) cancer, others not. They added five case studies of women who *did* develop breast cancer, but repeat the message that anyone contemplating ovarian stimulation for egg retrieval (this, importantly, also includes the growing number of young women who are told to freeze their egg cells for later use) must be told that the long-term adverse effects are not clearly established *because the studies have not been done.*

are hit when retrieving the egg cells. This has necessitated later blood transfusions if the bleeding remains unnoticed. It can also lead to bladder or even bowel injuries if the needle is inserted wrongly.

Viewing 'Eggsploitation' should be mandatory for anyone even thinking of using an egg 'donor' to fulfill their desire for an 'outsourced' child. This is especially important for gay men as they always need an egg donor. The question we all must ask is: how can anyone justify jeopardising a young woman's health and possibly life? How can such selfishness be publicly sanctioned by pro-surrogacy groups and, in some countries, the state?

And there are many more problems with this form of reproductive slavery. What is rarely mentioned is that throughout the preparatory phase, the three women involved undergo a roller coaster of emotions. The egg provider may curse the sickness and discomfort caused by the drugs that often severely interfere with her daily life and work, but, if she is paid between $US 5,000 and 10,000 (or more) per egg retrieval, as is customary in the USA, the prospect of good money will make her grit her teeth and ignore the pain. The 'surrogate' mother, already highly medicalised with daily injections and frequent ultrasounds to monitor the lining of her uterus and hormonal levels, is entering the next nine months of bondage where her life is not her own any more.

And what about the female partner of the commissioning couple who is not the egg donor? To the outside world she is a happy part of Team Baby when on the inside she might feel like a phenomenal failure: she should be the one getting pregnant, but she cannot. Selecting an egg provider by looking at porn-like photos of young beautiful women on the internet and 'choosing' the provider of half the genes of what will become 'her' child can unleash painful emotions that cause deep grief. And if she has any knowledge of the potential risks to the egg provider, her conscience about potentially injuring another woman might cause her sleepless nights.

If the embryo transfer is successful and a pregnancy starts, this brings many new challenges and potential health problems. Because the IVF clinic wants to insure that the commissioned baby will be free of 'defects', the pregnant woman has to submit to a battery of prenatal tests which may even lead to a mandated abortion, possibly against her own beliefs. If more than one embryo had been inserted and too many 'take', selective foetal pregnancy 'reduction' may be done. This entails the gruelling injection of potassium chloride (a salt) into the heart of one of the growing foetuses which then shrivels away in the womb next to the foetus(es) that are 'allowed' to continue to grow. This is difficult to envisage even for women who support a woman's right to abortion (as I do), but must be close to unbearable for a woman who is pro-life. Yet the contract the so-called surrogate signed mandates it. There may also be repair surgery on the foetus conducted in utero if the commissioning couple is determined to have a baby at any price.

It's one thing to write these lines: imagine if you were the woman in whose body such procedures are carried out?

The answer to such unwanted pain is *dissociation*. It is crucial that the pregnant woman is told again and again by her doctor, her counsellor (if she has one), family members, her partner – *until she internalises it herself* – that these growing cells in her uterus that are sustained by blood vessels she develops exclusively for this purpose in the placenta and which feed the developing baby nutrients including calcium from her bones *have nothing to do with her*, because she did not contribute her genes to this baby.

But genes are not the only bond between a mother and her baby. Few people know that even decades after her child is born, the birth mother still has a few of her or his cells in her body. Likewise, some of her own cells are passed on to her child (Dawe *et al.*, 2007).[18] And during pregnancy, so much else is shared as discussed in advice books for 'ordinary' pregnant women about the importance of stress, smoking, alcohol, certain foods and the moods of a pregnant woman including the type of music she listens to: all factors, we are told, that will influence the health and likes of the future child.[19]

---

18 In 'Cell Migration from Baby to Mother' (Gavin S Dawe *et al.* 2007), the authors describe how a small number of cells traffic across the placenta during the pregnancy and how "this exchange occurs both from the fetus to the mother (fetomaternal) and from the mother to the fetus."

19 Life before birth, now renamed 'foetal programming' or 'disease origins' is increasingly frequently examined. See for example, Thin Vo and Daniel B Hardy (2012) 'Molecular mechanisms underlying the fetal programming of adult diseases' <http://www.ncbi.nlm.nih.gov/pmc/articles/PMC3421023/>
Writing this makes me think of how many more avenues for control of pregnant 'surrogate' mothers there could be: commissioning couples who are Mozart or Stravinsky lovers might stipulate in the contract that she listen two hours each day to their favourite composer! As to food regulations, no

It is bizarre to hear commissioning couples proclaim that the baby growing in another woman's body is 'their' genetic child – even more so when they have used an egg donor who contributed half the nuclear genome (nDNA) to the developing child.

But it gets even more bizarre because every egg cell also includes mitochondrial DNA (mDNA): different and separate from nDNA. "Mitochondria are the energy-producing factories of the cell: without them a cell would not be able to generate energy from food" (Beekman, 2015).[20] And mDNA is passed on only via the mother; as Madeleine Beekman puts it: "Because all mitochondria you received come from your mother only, you are technically more related to your mum than to your dad." Your 'mum' in a surrogacy situation is the egg 'donor', your 'mother' is the birth mother in whose body the baby develops and swaps cells. Sperm donors beware: you are only half as important as you think you are.

A further nail in the coffin of the body deniers and gene lovers comes from India. As part of Indian ancient Ayurvedic culture, according to surrogacy researcher Sheela Saravanan

---

alcohol, no salt, no sugar might be the basics to start with, but no doubt many other forbidden foods might be added as well, including a host of recommended supplements. But how, exactly, do you forbid stress?

20 'Do you share more genes with your mother or your father?' <http://theconversation.com/do-you-share-more-genes-with-your-mother-or-your-father-50076?utm_medium=email&utm_campaign=The+Weekend+Conversation+-+3848&utm_content=The+Weekend+Conversation+-+3848+CID_61a7cc1a201fc294d7e8dd96475391da&utm_source=campaign_monitor&utm_term=Do%20you%20share%20more%20genes%20with%20your%20mother%20or%20your%20father>

(pers.com. June 2017): "Parturition and breastfeeding is considered a transfer of blood from the mother to the child and children are considered to be indebted to this and need to look after and have respect for their mothers all their life owing to this."

Amrita Pande, in her ethnography of India's surrogacy business (2015, p. 8) quotes a so-called surrogate mother, Parvati, who just underwent foetal reduction as saying:

> Doctor Madam told us that the babies wouldn't get enough space to move around and grow, so we should get the surgery. But both Nandini *didi* [the genetic mother] and I wanted to keep all three babies. I told Doctor Madam that I'll keep one and *didi* can keep two. *After all it's my blood even if it's their genes.* And who knows whether at my age I'll be able to have more babies (emphasis added by Pande).

Pande comments (2015, p. 8) that "Parvati, thus, uses her interpretation of the blood tie to make claims on the baby/fetus. Raveena makes a similar claim. But in addition to the substantial ties of blood, Raveena also emphasizes the labor of gestation and giving birth." Here is Pande's quote from Raveena (2015, p. 8):

> Anne [the genetic mother] wanted a girl but I told her even before the ultrasound, coming from me it will be a boy. My first two children were also boys. This one will be too. And see I was right, it is a boy! After all *they just gave the eggs, but the blood and all the sweat, all the effort is mine. Of course it's going after me* (emphasis added by Pande).

Amrita Pande adds (2015, p. 8): "This sweat (*paseena*) and the blood (*khoon*) tie between surrogate and fetus is often advocated by womb mothers as stronger than a connection based solely on genes.[21]

Indeed. Amrita Pande could have used these insights by pregnant 'surrogates' to make a plea for rejecting the international mantra "it's not my genes, it's not my baby" and advocate to stop surrogacy in India. Alas, instead, she comes up with some fictitious kinship ties, writing that

[T]he relationship between the two mothers – the womb mother [Pande's term] and the genetic or intended mother – is not merely competitive. Much like the kin ties forged with the baby, the ties with the intended mother allow womb mothers to cope with the emotional isolation and also challenge the medical construction of their relationship as merely contractual and easily disposable (2015, p. 9, my [] insertion).

Pande continues, "Deepa, another former surrogate, also believes her relationship with her client from Japan is based on mutual respect and reciprocity." But then a few lines later Pande concedes: "but ... relationships sustained beyond the contract period are rare. Most clients, apprehensive that the commercial surrogate will change her mind about giving the

---

21 For more on birth in Ayurvedic tradition, US Asian Studies Professor, Martha Selby (2005) writes about the way in which women's interior knowledge was incorporated into Sanskrit texts. The two competing powers are blood, provided by women, and semen, provided by men. In the Sanskrit tradition, in contrast to Ancient Greek medical ideas, "it is not the uterus that is the jug or pot: it is the whole woman herself; not just her womb, but the whole of her" (Selby 2005, p. 262).

baby away, prefer to sever all ties with her" and quotes another birth mother, Tejal, who feels very bitter about the way she was treated (2015, p. 9):

> There was a lot of problems with the delivery and I had to have 15–20 bottles of IV in just two days. Ultimately I got a scissor (Caesarian section). I was unconscious when the couple came and took away the baby. They didn't even show it to my husband. The baby would have been three years today. But I don't even know what he looks like. I used to think they would invite us to America. I used to think of her as a sister – *all of it went to waste*. Forget an invitation, they did not even call to see if we were dead or alive. The[y] just finished their business, picked up the baby and left (Pande's emphasis).

These are upsetting and sad tales from the surrogacy world. No doubt they are not isolated stories. In spite of this evidence, Amrita Pande is a strong supporter of surrogacy as 'work' and believes it is a woman's 'choice' (see Chapter 4, pp. 54–58 for further comments on Pande's research).

For those of us critical of surrogacy, the women's pain add feelings of sorrow about what so-called surrogate mothers endure, even if, or, especially when, their ancient culture tells them what their bodies know: that blood and sweat matter.

But to the brainwashed general public including the media (especially in rich westernised countries), the birth mother is a suitcase, an oven, in which a 'passenger' spends a few months until s/he plops out of the womb into the arms of their 'real' parent, their 'natural' father.[22] It is the 21st century's legacy of

---

22 A friend of mine who recently gave birth sent me a colour photo of her placenta. I wish I could reproduce it here because it shows the most amazing

the Homunculus theory promoted by Aristotle in the fourth century BCE when he assumed that a pregnant woman was but a vessel for the male sperm (formed in the brain!) which already contained a fully formed *male* human being![23]

Stripping both egg 'donor' and pregnant woman of their vital importance goes to the core of the dream of reproductive biologists to one day produce the motherless baby in an artificial womb. But until ectogenesis is perfected (see Conclusion, pp. 162–167 for more details), the real-life pregnant woman is so truly indoctrinated that she mostly agrees with the fallacy that this is not her child and happily calls herself a 'surrogate' – dissociation wins and post-modern writers such as Amrita Pande continue to play an important part in international discourses that call surrogacy 'work'.[24]

'tree' of blood vessels that connect the growing baby with its mother. As far as I know, suitcases don't have linings that can produce these sorts of formations!

23 Indeed Aristotle believed that women were deformities; a woman was an abnormality when the male development had gone wrong (see Garr, 2012 p. 159).

24 Postmodernism came to be very fashionable in the 1980s/1990s in academia where it morphed into the philosophy 'du jour' for (not) explaining many social problems. In postmodern thinking, there is no truth, nothing is real and there are multiple subjectivities that can be conjured up to explain or describe a state of being. It is hugely responsible for the increasing state of dissociation that the world has adopted. Think climate change deniers, the assumed necessity of war, the 'choice' of prostitution, the medicalisation of the masses, etc. See Somer Brodribb's excellent exposé *Nothing Mat(t)ers* (1992). I have strongly critiqued postmodern thinking, see Klein (1996) in *Radically Speaking*, Bell and Klein (eds.) which also includes a whole section of radical feminist critiques of postmodernism.

Going back to the events in a 'surrogate' mother's journey, giving birth usually marks the beginning of a new human being's entrance into their mother's life. Sadly, in the context of surrogacy, it is *the end* of their relationship forged over nine months. If an egg 'donor' was involved, in the weeks leading up to the birth, pre-eclampsia, a high blood pressure condition that can be life-threatening for the baby and the pregnant woman can occur (see Elenis *et al.*, 2015; Masoudian *et al.*, 2016). Placenta praevia is another serious condition more frequent with 'donor' eggs. The placenta has moved down in the womb and become attached to the uterus just above the cervix. As the baby grows and presses downwards, haemorrhaging often occurs. This is also very dangerous for both baby and mother and long bed rest, in order to keep still, is the only remedy (see Chapter 6, pp. 122–137 on a sister surrogacy in Australia where the birth mother was confined to bed for seven weeks). Finally, placental abruption can happen in which the placenta detaches itself from the uterine wall, also more frequent in pregnancies when donor eggs are used. All of these conditions need weeks of bed rest and experienced obstetricians to deal with them so that both baby and mother do not come to harm. Are women who are contemplating being 'surrogates' with 'donor' eggs told about these potential serious pregnancy conditions before they sign any papers? How does this relate to the question of whether surrogacy is a 'choice'?

In many cases the baby is born prematurely, often via a Caesarian section.[25] This means, as we have seen above in Tejal's story from India (see p. 27), that the birthing woman is anaesthetised and may not get to see her baby. What she is left with is a heavy heart and breasts full of milk. But as she has been indoctrinated to consider this baby her great act of kindness for a deserving couple, this is what she is trying to tell herself while blocking out whatever bond she may feel with the baby. But for some women (not all), this denial will re-surface as post-partum depression, pain, regret, or anger, followed by severe depression and despair, often years later (see Elizabeth Kane's story, Chapter 6, pp. 112–116).

And the 'other woman', the female partner of a heterosexual commissioning couple is now in charge of a tiny newborn that, as is well known, posits many challenges for any new mother looking after her baby/ies. Indeed, s/he may bring her to the brink of a nervous breakdown as she is trying to be the perfect mother to this foreign being that suffers from colic, doesn't stop crying, and won't let her sleep for months. But to the outside world she has to be radiant with happiness: after all, she and her partner finally have 'their' much longed-for child. Question: since the 'surrogate' was told again and again that her birth child is not her baby, as it does not have 'her genes', is the 'social mother' told the same lie? I assume not. This is just one

---

25 In November 2015, the *World Journal of Obstetrics and Gynecology* (WJOG) published an important paper on outcomes of 'surrogate' pregnancies in California (Nicolau *et al.*, 2015). The authors found that "Surrogate pregnancies result in higher maternity and newborn costs with increased rates of multiple births and creates a moral hazard for hospitals" (p. 2).

example of the many contradictory fibs in the tales from the surrogacy world.

The fact that some women feel resentful about the baby they know is not their own, and bitter, because they remain infertile, is not allowed to be talked about in public. In her memoir *Birth Mother* (1988/1990), America's first 'surrogate', Elizabeth Kane whose real name is Mary Beth, writes about Margo, the commissioning mother, who shortly after the birth of Justin quipped "if there's ever another baby in this house, it's coming out of my body." That never happened; in spite of years of trying, she remained infertile. See Chapter 6, pp. 112–116 for more on Kane's remarkable story including her sad, but astute, comment that

> [S]urrogate motherhood is nothing more than the transference of pain from one woman to another. One woman is in anguish because she cannot become a mother, and another woman – such as myself – may suffer for the rest of her life because she cannot know the child she bore for someone else (1988/1990, p. 272).

Knowing all of this should surely make it impossible to talk about 'rights', 'choices' and 'agency'. And yet the pro-surrogacy brigade persists.

In the next chapter, I will consider the situation of children born from surrogacy arrangements and compare them to (forced) adoption practices of the past.

Chapter 3
What of the children born from surrogacy?

Whenever we hear of children being separated from their mother or parents, most people express sorrow and/or anger, depending on the situation. We feel indignant when we hear that Bokum Harum in Nigeria kidnaps girls and forces them into sexual slavery aimed at bearing children to increase their population. Similarly, we are profoundly upset by tales of Daesh fighters kidnapping and raping young Christian, Shiite and Yazidi girls. We are outraged when we hear of recurring scandals such as overseas adoption of so-called orphans that is later revealed as a scam in which babies are bought for a pittance from poor mothers. We are even more outraged when we hear of girls trafficked into prostitution which is widespread in India and Sri Lanka and other poor nations such as Bangladesh where destitute single women are offered a hospital bed to give birth to their babies who are then sold as sex slaves to Saudi Arabia (pers. comm. Farida Akhter, 2005). We condemn in strong words the past practices in Australia of removing Indigenous children from their parents which we know as The Stolen Generations. Or coercing unwed white women to give up their babies during the 20th century up to the 1980s 'for their own good' to a 'proper' family which was to provide for them far better than their birth mother – the 'fallen' single woman – ever could (see more below).

But somehow, when the practice of surrogacy is discussed, these social norms appear to fall by the wayside. Again and again we hear that people seeking to obtain a child via surrogacy were 'desperate' to start a family and 'heartbroken' that *their* desire for a child could not be 'naturally' fulfilled. To put it differently, it seems that many people condone – or indeed encourage – what is, quite simply the scenario of a pay-as-you-go product child which in this world of entitlement is made to order for those who are rich enough to afford it. The newborn babies in this origin story have no say in the matter; they are seen as blank canvases whose lives start at the moment when they are lifted out of the 'incubator's' womb in a Caesarean section. It is the commissioning couple – gay or straight – who will now guide them through the steps of becoming children and then adults.

It is, unashamedly, an adult- or parent-centred view, with the basic human rights of newborn babies ignored. Surrogacy is not only a benign neoliberal fantasy, but being pregnant with someone else's embryo is seen as 'work' (see also Chapter 4, pp. 52–66). As *Forbes Magazine* blithely pronounced: "You'd rent a nanny or a house painter. Why not rent a uterus?" (Smith, 2013). It is also deeply patriarchal: the vessel carrying and birthing the child does not matter. She can be ignored. It is a retelling of the old myth that it is storks who bring babies, never to be seen or heard of again once they have dropped the child down the chimney.

Such glib thinking fuelled by postmodern ideology contrasts with the large number of authors who believe that as babies develop in their mother's womb, in tandem with growing bones and tissue as well as nerve and muscle cells (as I discussed in Chapter 2), they also 'grow' spirits and souls. And who posit that these developments are profoundly influenced by emotions experienced by the pregnant woman – be they joyful or stressful – as the nutrients in her blood grow her child from an embryo to a small person ready to enter this world. A type of psychoanalysis referred to as 'regression therapy' focuses on this time in the womb and, often with the help of hypnotherapy, aims to explore the inner life of a grown-up person by going back to especially important (or hurtful) times in their life, such as when they grew a baby in their bodies that they then gave away (see IBRT, no date).

But also contrast the facile story of happy-go-lucky surrogacy with thousands of stories from adopted children who felt they never really belonged to their adoptive families in spite of being cared for and loved deeply (see Mackieson, 2015). And who looked for their birth mother and sperm donor for decades, often to be disappointed when, as adults, they finally receive their birth records only to discover that their mother or father was already dead. Or, even if they did manage to find and meet their birth mother, and it is a good reunion, endure on-going grief and feelings of regrets over a life that did not include their birth brothers and sisters.

As Penny Mackieson stated (pers. comm., 2014) :

> As an adoptee from birth affected by Australia's past coercive adoption practices, it saddens me that pro-surrogacy proponents do not appreciate the lifelong difficulties for the children of not being able to know about and/or have ongoing relationships with the parents who created and gestated them – irrespective of how well loved and parented we have been/are by our social parents. It is obvious to me that the added dimension of having been conceived and born through a commercial contract involving the exchange of money would create even more ongoing challenges for the person's identity, self worth and psychological health throughout their life.

And as relinquishing mother, Jo Fraser, points out in her Submission to the Australian Surrogacy Inquiry (2016, p. 3):

> The consequences of being adopted for many are that they feel that they were traded as a powerless commodity, and can result in low self-esteem and a sense of rejection and worthlessness. Imagine how much this is exacerbated if the relinquishment, or trading, of the child is premeditated and carefully planned in fine detail?
>
> The bottom line is that, wherever the surrogacy occurs—whether it is here or overseas—and however well or badly it is done, what we are doing is reasserting the idea that children are the property of adults and we are buying babies. Just because we want something desperately does not mean we have the right to have it.

And Catherine Lynch, in her 2016 Submission for the Australian Adoptee Rights Action Group to the Australian Surrogacy Inquiry states (2016, p. 3):

> As adoptees we say: the loss of the mother's body at birth is experienced as a trauma which is felt at first as an inexpressible loss (what can the baby do but cry?) and creates a lacuna of despair

that never leaves the person despite a lifetime of adaptation and socialisation, and despite the fact that, this trauma having occurred before the development of long-term memory, the trauma is not consciously 'remembered'. The experience of loss of part of the self, the mother whom the child seeks after birth, is not somehow left behind because the baby is unable to retain its mental image.

Indeed, these comments from both adoptees and relinquishing mothers do beg the question: *why are we committing such fraud yet again?* Have we not learned anything from the lessons of the past? In Australia, on 13 February 2008, then Prime Minister Kevin Rudd presented a moving National Apology to the Stolen Generations of Australia's Indigenous peoples. And on 21 March 2013, then Prime Minister Julia Gillard offered a heartfelt National Apology Speech including the National Apology for Forced Adoptions (Gillard, 2013) to the (white) mothers of the 250,000 removed babies (Lynch, 2016). Here are some excerpts from her speech:

> Too often they did not see their baby's face. They could not soothe their baby's first cries, never felt their baby's warmth or smelt their baby's skin. They could not give their own baby a name. These babies grew up with other names and in other homes, creating a sense of abandonment and loss that sometimes could never be made whole.
>
> Today, this parliament, on behalf of the Australian people, takes responsibility and apologises for the policies and practices that forced the separation of mothers from their babies, which created a lifelong legacy of pain and suffering.
>
> And we recognise the hurt these actions caused to brothers and sisters, grandparents, partners and extended family members.

We deplore the shameful practices that denied you, the mothers, your fundamental rights and responsibilities to love and care for your children. You were not legally or socially acknowledged as their mothers. And you were yourselves deprived of care and support.

We resolve, as a nation, to do all in our power to make sure these practices are never repeated. In facing future challenges, we will remember the lessons of family separation. Our focus will be on protecting the fundamental rights of children and on the importance of the child's right to know and be cared for by his or her parents (my emphasis).[26]

I quote from this speech at length, because it is disappointing that after Prime Minister Gillard's profound words that were widely discussed and generally welcomed, the Commonwealth of Australia does not wholeheartedly reject surrogacy. Nor are people who travel overseas for commercial surrogacy charged if they live in New South Wales, Queensland or the Australian Territory where this constitutes a crime. (In Chapter 5 I will discuss the 2016 Australian Parliamentary Inquiry into Surrogacy.)

Finally, it is good to know that some children who were born via surrogacy in the 1980s are now speaking out.[27]

Thirty-year old Jessica Kern campaigns to outlaw surrogacy and said to the *New York Post*: "Like I would choose this for

---

26 Julia Gillard's speech is included as Appendix 1 in Penny Mackieson's 2015 book *Adoption Deception: A Personal and Professional Journey* (pp. 151–159).

27 Another misnomer is beginning to appear in news reports on surrogacy: that of 'the surrogate child'. Of course there is nothing 'surrogate' about a child born of a surrogacy arrangement: she or he is a real as any of us.

myself? When the only reason you're in this world is a big fat paycheck, it's degrading."[28] And 'Brian' writes on his blog Son of a Surrogate: "Yes I am angry. Yes I feel cheated ... It's a shame and it sucks for me. Hell it sucks for all of us." And "How do you think we feel about being created specifically to be given away? You should all know that kids form their own opinions."[29]

Other children born of surrogacy may never get their voices heard. They are those deemed 'deficient' because they were products of reproductive technology tourism born with a disability that was not detected in prenatal tests.[30]

Abandoned by their commissioning parents who did not order 'damaged goods', these white babies disappear in Indian or Thai orphanages and are never heard from again. The inspiring story of Pattharamon Chanbua who insisted on keeping Baby Gammy[31] who was born with Down syndrome and rejected by his parents who only took his able-bodied sister back to Australia, is an exception.[32]

---

28 <http://nypost.com/2014/06/16/children-of-surrogacy-campaign-to-outlaw-the-practice/>

29 Brian is indeed one angry young man. It is definitely worth reading his blog; <http://sonofasurrogate.tripod.com/>

30 As Sanoj Rajan, Professor in the School of Law of Ansal University in India discusses, the problems for these children born with disabilities through surrogacy is often compounded by 'statelessness' as the intended parents refuse to take the child. See <http://www.institutesi.org/worldsstateless17.pdf> for references to some of these cases.

31 'Thai surrogate baby Gammy: Australian parents contacted', 7 August 2014; <http://www.bbc.com/news/world-asia-28686114>

32 In an ABC TV 7.30 News report on 29 June 2017, Baby Gammy – now called Grammy – is seen as a happy three-year-old, doing very well in Kinder-

Pattharamon Chanbua also tried to get custody of her daughter Pipah whom she wanted to come and live with her and her twin brother Gammy. But in April 2016, an Australian judge, Justice Stephen Thackray turned Chanbua's application down on the grounds that Pipah had lived in Australia for all her life: a mere sixteen months (Safi, 14 April 2016). In other words, a convicted paedophile – the commissioning father – has more rights than a birth mother – Father Rights triumph yet again!

Lastly, what must be mentioned also is the deeply disturbing fact that the practice of surrogacy lets a sexual predator *order* babies that he can then abuse.

Shortly after the Baby Gammy story, we were told of another unconscionable tale, also from Thailand. As Samantha Hawley reported (2 September 2014): "An Australian who fathered surrogate twins with a Thai woman has been charged with sexually abusing the children." The heterosexual man was also charged with child pornography which was found in a raid on his home. His wife denied any knowledge of abusive acts. She says that not long after the couple had returned from Thailand with the twins, her husband lost his job. The marriage broke down – he allegedly had a violent temper – and the twins now live with his ex-wife.

Meanwhile the birth mother in Thailand felt so bad about these events that she wants her children back (she used her own eggs so she is also their genetic mother). But at the time of reporting, the children remained in Australia as they did not

---

garten. However, his mother worries that the $240,000 in the trust fund established for Gammy by Australian donors will only last two more years.

know that they were half Thai and did not speak a single word of Thai. The birth mother Siriwan Nitichad had received $5,500.

An earlier story about child sexual abuse, where two men bought a baby from a Russian mother for $8,000 in 2005, is bone chilling. These two men, Australian citizen Mark J. Newton and his long-term US boyfriend, Peter Truong, were interviewed in 2010 by a local ABC reporter from Far North Queensland (they were living in Cairns) and celebrated as gay dads, before, due to an ongoing underground police investigation, they were arrested in February 2011 as part of an international paedophile ring. Not only was their son abused by his two 'fathers' virtually from birth (a video was found in which Newton performed a sex act on the boy before he was two weeks' old, but flown overseas and sexually abused in group sessions of paedophiles for over six years. Amongst them were members of the 'Boy Lovers Network'. It is difficult to see how this boy can ever recover from such early trauma, which it seems he was groomed to think of as 'normal'. Newton was sentenced to 40 years' and Truong to 30 years' prison (Ralston, 30 June 2013).

Of course, we all hope that such dismal stories are rare and that most commissioning parents, straight or gay, are decent human beings even if misguided by a narcissistic desire for 'their' own baby. But how do we know for sure? In our neoliberal globalised world in which, when one surrogacy market closes, another opens, and greed is the motive for their existence, how can we be sure that such abuses do not happen far more frequently that we are made aware of? There are probably many tales to tell of children born of surrogacy who were later caught up in bitter divorces with one or both parents rejecting them as 'not my child'. They might be forgiven for feeling like 'damaged goods' and the search for their birth mother – and egg 'donor' – may take them on an often illusionary, and deeply painful journey.

There is also significant harm done to the other children of 'surrogate' mothers. The US first ever commercial 'surrogate', Elizabeth Kane, had been willing and enthusiastic in 1980, but drastically changed her view on surrogacy later. One of the reasons for the change was the effect of the surrogacy on her children. Her teenage daughter was mercilessly teased at school when front page pictures of her mother appeared in yet another newspaper or on TV, and frequently came home in tears. Then she withdrew from her family. And Elizabeth found her other daughter sitting at breakfast one day and sobbing, "I never got to hold my baby brother." Her son, who was only four years' old at the time, when watching a TV program showing the birth, began screaming "Mama's baby all gone. Mama's baby all gone." At thirteen years he "... is in a self contained special education classroom for learning-disabled children. He is still a clinging, fearful child" (all quotes from Kane, 1988/90, pp. 252–257, see Chapter 6, pp. 112–116 for more information). When another US woman, Nancy Barass, who had been a 'surrogate' in California, came home from hospital, her daughter, aged eight at the time, asked: "Mummy, if I am a bad girl, are you going to give me away too?" (in Klein, 1989b, p. 158).

These are such sad stories and the international literature on surrogacy is littered with them. Elizabeth Kane's and Nancy

Barass' experiences were in the 1980s. Why, 30 years later, are we still pretending surrogacy is a wonderful thing? And why do we have to be confronted with headlines like these: 'Carrying a child for someone else should be celebrated – and paid' (Editorial, *The Economist*, 13 May 2017).

Based on our knowledge of traumatic experiences with hundreds of thousands of stolen children from Indigenous and white women alike, whose adoptions were often misguided and caused deep harm to all parties involved, I strongly believe there is just one answer to the latest practice of separating children from the women who gave birth to them: Stop Surrogacy Now.[33]

Mothers who were forced to give their children away in the 1960s and 1970s, and Aboriginal women whose children were stolen over many generations, are on side in opposing surrogacy. So are so-called 'donor' offspring: children created with anonymous sperm or eggs, some of whom are now on a life-long quest to find who they are related to.[34]

I ask, how can we have forgotten the many heartbreaking stories from adoption, both from relinquishing mothers and adopted children, now adults? For those of us in Australia, did we not hear former Prime Minister Julia Gillard's heartfelt apology

---

33 Stop Surrogacy Now (SSN) is an international activist campaign that was started in May 2015. See Chapter 6, pp. 145–153 for information on the many inspiring SSN actions; <http://www.stopsurrogacynow.com>

34 In Australia, the organisation Tangled Web is a powerful lobby group to reverse anonymity granted to sperm donors in the 1960s and 1970s so that donor sperm adults might still have a chance to meet the man who fathered them. See Lauren Burns' story to track down her donor father at <http://www.abc.net.au/austory/content/2014/s4065081.htm>

to these women and their children? Why are we repeating these mistakes, and why are we not even talking about it but instead pretend that surrogacy is just a modern way of making babies and there is nothing wrong with it? Why do we not concede that the 'product child' as tradable commodity has never consented to being a 'take-away baby': removed from their birth mother and given to strangers, aka 'intended parents'? Why, in fact do we not officially call surrogacy 'child trafficking' and 'child buying' because this is precisely what we do to these babies.[35] The acceptance of surrogacy will lead to a new generation of grieving women, and of children who mourn their unknown birth mother (and egg 'donor'). And we should not be surprised if there is another Australian inquiry in a few decades' time – and another apology to children who were 'given away'.

Or could there be a different story? In the next chapter, I will explore if surrogacy can be ethical.

---

35 Swedish author, Kajsa Ekis Ekman, asks this pertinent question in her insightful book *Being and Being Bought: Prostitution, Surrogacy and the Split Self* (2013, pp. 144–147).

Chapter 4
Can surrogacy be ethical?

After the story broke in May 2014 that Baby Gammy had been left behind in Thailand by his Australian commissioning parents and was now cared for by his birth mother Pattharamon Chanbua (see also p. 1 and p. 39), an intense media debate began in Australia aimed at making the case for allowing commercial surrogacy.[36] This campaign was spearheaded by a very organised pro-surrogacy lobby consisting of IVF clinics and consumer groups such as Surrogacy Australia and Families Through Surrogacy, and supported by some legal academics and the head of the Family Court, Chief Justice Diana Bryant (Feneley, 30 April 2015). As a result, print and TV media, on the whole, presented surrogacy as a feel-good story: desperate couples, gay and straight, longing to have their own child, and cute little babies in designer clothes leading a happy life with extremely well-off parents.[37] It was much harder to get an alternative

---

36 At the time of going to print, July 2017, commercial surrogacy remains prohibited as the Australian government has still not responded to the 2016 report 'Surrogacy Matters' following a Government Inquiry; see Chapter 5, pp. 73–86 for more details on this Inquiry.

37 See ABC-TV's *Four Corners* program, which on 22 September 2014 aired an episode called 'Made in Thailand' which highlighted some of the

viewpoint published with only few of us succeeding (Allan, 4 August 2014; Klein, 20 August 2014).

Unfortunately, despite the deeply problematic Baby Gammy story in terms of exploiting women in developing countries and eugenics implicit in surrogacy when 'imperfect' babies are born that are then rejected by the baby buyers, the central question in print and TV media was not whether surrogacy should be endorsed at all, but instead, how surrogacy could be made 'better'. Central to this emphasis was the question of whether commercial surrogacy should be legalised in Australia where it could then be well regulated and, as Justice Bryant suggested, could be 'ethical' (Brennan, 18 April 2015).

Proponents of this view included surrogacy user Sam Everingham who is the father of two girls that he and his partner commissioned in India.[38] Everingham founded the consumer lobby group Surrogacy Australia in 2010 and remains heavily involved as Global Director of Families Through Surrogacy

---

ethical dilemmas; <http://www.abc.net.au/4corners/stories/2014/09/22/4090232.htm>

38 Sam Everingham's first attempt at surrogacy in India ended with the pregnant woman suffering a miscarriage of her twin boys. One baby survived, but died a few weeks later. To make sure there would at least be one child in the next round, Everingham and his partner hired two Indian 'surrogates' and each man contributed his sperm to multiple embryos that were then implanted in the two women. As too many embryos developed, the two *men* agreed to so-called 'foetal reduction'. Journalist Julia Medew tells us that the experience "led to more trauma" for Everingham and his partner (Medew, 2013)? But what about the 'trauma' of the two pregnant women? After the 'foetal reductions', two healthy girls were born in 2011.

which organises high-profile conferences in Australia, the USA, Sweden, Ireland and the UK for prospective surrogacy users.[39]

Following on from Justice Bryant's well-publicised statements earlier in April, on 14 May 2015, the *Sydney Morning Herald* conducted a so-called 'debate' on whether commercial surrogacy was ethical and should be permitted in Australia. Sam Everingham put the case for the 'yes' side and made the tantalising suggestion that if we changed our language, commercial surrogacy that was 'ethical' would be possible. In his words (Everingham/Tobin, 2014):

> In the US, where ethical surrogacy has been practised for more than 30 years, the woman carrying a child for the intended parent is referred to as a gestational carrier rather than a surrogate mother.

---

39 I attended the Third Families Through Surrogacy Conference in Melbourne, 24–25 May 2014, advertised as "It's on again. The largest event globally for intended parents and surrogates." Present were eight IVF clinics from Australia, the USA (California) and India; six Australian legal firms; so-called surrogacy 'facilitators' and agencies from the USA, Thailand, Mexico and Eastern Europe and beaming surrogacy parents, babies in tow. And there were good looking 'surrogates' and egg 'donors' and a beautiful Tree of Life logo for the inner sanctum: a closed Forum for prospective baby buyers. The atmosphere was one of wholesome joy and excitement: your baby journey begins now. No criticism was allowed. When an academic dared to mention just a few problems with surrogacy in India (while repeatedly asserting how totally she supported surrogacy), she was rudely criticised by a man in the audience who claimed everything she had just said was wrong and stupid. I tried to find her in the lunch break but she must have fled. After two days, I left bedazzled by so much exciting potential. Many glossy brochures, a 'Handbook from the Third Australian *Consumer* Conference' (my emphasis) and a handful of stylish pens in hand ensured I would not forget this event for a long time. As a friend who attended put it: "it was like swimming through asbestos." We opted for a drink afterwards instead of a cold shower.

There is sound reasoning for this – they are not a 'replacement' mother. While the research shows children born through surrogacy understand this from a young age, wider Australian society does not. Our language reinforces this error.

He concedes that "not all surrogacy is carried out ethically, but remedying that is a matter of properly funded education, psychological support, counselling and compensation." His urgent advice for Australian lawmakers is to 'get on with it', start a national inquiry and then bring in laws that allow commercial surrogacy.

Three points in his statement need discussion. The first is that to call surrogacy as practised in the USA for more than 30 years 'ethical' is either revealing his deep ignorance about past and current events in the USA, and/or repeating glowing statements made by Californian IVF doctors who are always welcomed panelists at the annual Australian conferences of Families through Surrogacy. As I will elaborate further in Chapter 6 (pp. 103–110, also pp. 148–149), surrogacy practices in the USA have been criticised by radical feminists since the early 1980s as exploitative (see Klein, 1989b; Rowland, 1992; Raymond, 1993/1995) and this criticism continues today (Lahl, 2016).

Secondly, his idea that the solution to problems with surrogacy is to name a human being called 'woman' who grows a baby for nine months in her body and then gives birth to it, a 'gestational carrier' shows his, and many other pro-surrogacy supporters' abysmal lack of understanding of, and respect for, women.

Thirdly, the phrase 'gestational carrier' erases women

(biological females who have two XX sex chromosomes) as the only living human beings who can grow and bear babies.[40] It also negates the inevitable relationship a pregnant woman develops with her developing child.

I suggest such sexist pronouncements are deeply unethical.

Representing the counter argument in this 'debate', Bernadette Tobin, who is the Director of the Plunkett Centre for Ethics at St Vincent's Hospital and the Australian Catholic University, responded with a resounding *No* (Everingham/ Tobin, 2014):

> Surrogacy intentionally violates a child's entitlement to be brought up – if at all possible – by his or her natural parents. Surrogacy intentionally violates the gestational link between the child and the natural mother. No surrogacy contract can protect the child from the wrong done to him or her by being brought into the world in these circumstances, whether or not money changes hands.

And further: "If we thought that by legalising commercial surrogacy in Australia we could give surrogacy an ethically sound underpinning we would be deceiving ourselves."[41]

---

40 So-called male-to-female transgender activists would like this to change and have asked for the UK National Health Service (NHS) to pay for 'womb transplants' into 'women' born as boys. Feminist activist, UK journalist Julie Bindel, called such demands "a twisted notion as to what constitutes a 'real' woman (3 July 2017, *Deccan Chronicle*). To date, only a handful of babies have been born with the help of womb transplants in Sweden into *women* who had no uterus. Transferring a uterus into a male body, and expecting it to work, reflects a typical patriarchal reduction of what a biologically female body is actually capable of doing.

41 Bernadette Tobin had already expressed similar doubts about both commercial and so-called altruistic surrogacy in *The Age* on 20 April 2015.

To continue with the discussion of whether surrogacy can be 'ethical', we also need to analyse the image that the pro-surrogacy lobby – and the mainstream media – constructs of the women who act as so-called surrogate mothers.

Swedish author and journalist, Kajsa Ekis Ekman, has authored a book that compares prostitution and surrogacy. Discussing the media perception of what kind of a woman is a 'good' surrogate mother, based on her research of British and US surrogate forums such as surromomsonline.com, Ekman writes in *Being and Being Bought: Prostitution, Surrogacy and the Split Self*: "They emphasize their generosity, talk of wanting to help, of heeding a call" (2013, p. 177). She quotes from surrogacy advocate's Betsy Aigen's *Motivations of Surrogate Mothers* (1996) in which Aigen claims that "being a surrogate is a life experience that allows some women real success in altering their emotional state in a direction they desire and fulfilling ideal images of themselves" (2013, p. 177).

What does this say about the most prized attributes a woman should display: being kind, nurturing and giving, and putting others first to the detriment of her own psychological well being and physiological health? Clearly this dissociation, this 'Split Self' – as Ekman calls it – can take a terrible toll.

Announcing the start of the global Stop Surrogacy Now campaign in May 2015 on the ABC's Religion and Ethic website, I asked the same question – Can Surrogacy be Ethical? – responding with the suggestion to "... call out this cruel business for what it is: trafficking in babies; reproductive slavery; a violation of the human rights of both the birth mother and her offspring" (Klein, 18 May 2015b).

Becoming a 'surrogate', for some women, can also be a result of trying to 'atone' for what they did previously in their lives: whether it was an abortion, or giving a child up for adoption. Being a 'surrogate', according to therapist and author, Phyllis Chesler, "... is, for many, a way to cleanse themselves of guilt and shame" (in Ekman, p. 182). Indeed, as Ekman writes, being a 'surrogate' can be an attempt to numb the pain by repeating this experience not just once, but multiple times: "Many surrogates describe a mixture of grief, longing, guilt and emptiness. The solution is often to go through the whole procedure again" (2013, p. 183).

But as Ekman continues: "It becomes a never-ending circle of losses, where the woman recreates the feeling of wholeness with the child she lost just to lose it again and start over from the beginning" (p. 183).

Should we really encourage women to inflict such pain on themselves, and do it all under the guise of being a loving, kind and caring individual who wants to help? From early childhood, girls are encouraged to put others first, so acting out of 'love' for others' unmet desires feeds right into the exploitative discourse of the pro-surrogacy lobby who fall over themselves praising women as 'angels' who bestow the gift of life – a baby – to desperately sad couples.

If we think back to the question of 'choice' (as earlier mentioned in Chapter 2, pp. 16–19), when society at large rewards women for putting others first – to the detriment of our well being – can we call this 'choice', free will, or 'agency'? I find it particularly distressing to read about the many tales of 'surrogate' mothers who were showered with presents, taken on holidays and talked to every day before and during the time of their pregnancy – only to be dumped after the baby was born. Still, carrying on as martyrs, and calling it their 'choice', sadly, earns high praise in a patriarchal society. As one birth mother recalls (in Ekman, p. 182):

> I had a rough delivery, a C-section, and my lung collapsed because I had the flu, but it was worth every minute of it. If I were to die from childbirth, that's the best way to die. You died for a cause, a good one.

Surely, such self-defeating behaviour should not be praised but discouraged wherever possible in the strongest possible terms. How does this woman assume her 'own' children react when they hear her utter these lines? Do they see her as a shining example of the self-less heroines they have encountered in patriarchal fairy tales – or as an uncaring human being that would 'choose' to leave them motherless in order to fulfill a loftier goal?

Those who maintain that surrogacy can be 'ethical' should not promote such behaviour which, quite simply, is toxic for women, both as individuals and members of the sex class women.

But many poor women become surrogates out of necessity and this leads us to the question of whether surrogacy should be considered 'work'. And if we considered it as work, could it then be made 'ethical'? As Andrea Dworkin pointed out in 1983 (p. 182):

> ... the state has constructed the social, economic, and political situation in which the sale of some sexual or reproductive capacity

is necessary to the survival of women; and yet the selling is seen to be an act of individual will – the only kind of assertion of individual will in women that is vigorously defended as a matter of course by most of those who pontificate about female freedom ... The individual woman is a fiction – as is her will – since individuality is precisely what women are denied when they are defined and used as a sex class.

So, what if we decided to call surrogacy work that could be used to give the sex class women, and especially poor women, a better chance to survive the harsh and unfair economic realities in which they find themselves? Kyle Smith, writing in *Forbes Magazine* (3 October, 2013), believes it is a no brainer. After a visit to well known fertility specialist Dr Nayana Patel's surrogacy clinic in Anand, Gujarat (a poor state in India), he opines:

Dr. Patel chafes at suggestions that what she is overseeing is a 'baby factory'. But of course that's what she's doing. And it's perfectly fine, a big win for everyone involved ... a new and innovative marketplace that brings together willing buyers and sellers.

Smith further notes that

most Westerners wouldn't raise an eyebrow if Patel's women came to the US to clean their toilets for a minimum wage (or maybe less, if they happened to be illegal immigrants). How is giving these same women a huge sum (to them) to carry a fetus unconscionable?

Kyle Smith's crass equation of cleaning toilets with growing/ birthing a baby, and bringing together "willing buyers and sellers" may appear 'vulgar' to some pro-surrogacy supporters who prefer to talk about 'ethical' surrogacy. But like it or not, if surrogacy is to be defined as work, then such equations have to be seen as a fair comment.

The case for defining commercial surrogacy as work and then use labour laws to supposedly make it fair and equitable – Fair Trade Surrogacy (drawing on medical practitioner, Casey Humbyrd's, 2009 proposition) – is made by a number of writers, amongst them sociologist Amrita Pande. Pande, working in South Africa, sees herself as an authority on surrogacy due to her ten years of ethnographic research with 'womb mothers' (her term) in India (see e.g. *Wombs in Labor: Transnational Commercial Surrogacy in India,* Pande, 2014; but also Pande 2015; 2016 and 2017).

Pande locates surrogacy – which she also refers to as 'contract pregnancy' – within the extensive informal labour market in India. She sees surrogacy as a 'choice' (albeit among a limited range of options), likens it to domestic work and 'sex work' and wants it to be well regulated by labour laws and standards.

She is highly critical of countries – now including India – that aim to end surrogacy by banning commercial surrogacy, because of "the utter naivety of trying to resolve a global problem merely through restrictive national legislations" (2017, p. 328),[42] but also because

> ... commercial surrogacy becomes a powerful challenge to the age-old dichotomy constructed between production and reproduction.

---

42 Amrita Pande appears to overlook that only a handful of countries allow commercial surrogacy (e.g. eight states plus Washington DC in the USA, Ukraine, Russia, Georgia). In other words, having laws prohibiting surrogacy is not the exception, but the rule.

Women's reproductive capacities are valued and monetized outside of the so-called private sphere. *As commercial surrogates, women use their bodies, wombs and sometimes breasts, as instruments of labour* (2015, p. 12, my emphasis).

However, before those of us opposed to surrogacy have time to pick our 'instruments of labours' off the floor, she contradicts her own statement by continuing:

But just as commercial surrogacy subverts these gendered dichotomies, it simultaneously reifies them. When reproductive bodies of women become the only source, requirement and product of a labour market, and fertility becomes the only asset women can use to earn wages, women essentially *get reduced to their reproductive capacities, ultimately reifying their historically constructed role in the gender division of labour* (2015, p. 12, my emphasis).

This is an excellent and pretty uncontestable statement with which most feminists of whatever 'variety' and wherever they live in the world, would agree. And a great argument against surrogacy! It is indeed one of the reasons why commodifying womb mothers' bodies and souls as 'work' is the wrong way to go in a deeply patriarchal state such as India (and elsewhere as well). Much needed poverty reduction for billions of disenfranchised and illiterate women who suffer all sorts of economic and social discrimination cannot be alleviated through the sale or rent of these female bodies themselves: not in sexual and not in reproductive prostitution. Nor can the trafficking in, and sale of, babies constitute an ethical way of pulling a small number of women and their families out of poverty.

But because Pande wants to have it both ways, we are left wandering in the post-modern haze of the day, wondering what she will say next.

The globalised neo-liberal marketplace ideology wins. Amrita Pande's commitment to surrogacy as work overrides her concerns about its patriarchal reification of women 'as nature'. She is intent on bestowing 'agency' to womb mothers in developing countries instead of seeing them as victims as she purports abolitionists do with our eurocentric and 'moralising' judgments.[43] Sadly, she ignores the many-faceted harms that surrogacy entails.

She also invokes the 'moral panic' argument, supposedly stemming from 'anxiety that reached panic levels' which led governments in Thailand, Nepal, Cambodia and the state of Tabasco in Mexico to prohibit commercial surrogacy (2016, p. 1). As a consequence, she opposes the Surrogacy (Regulation) Bill that was approved by the Indian Union Cabinet on 24 August, 2016.[44] Based on the British guidelines by the Human

---

43 Pande uses the term 'eurocentric' to dismiss early predictions in the 1980s by Andrea Dworkin, Gena Corea and Barbara Katz Rothman that in the future, birth mothers might be kept in 'reproductive brothels' in third world countries. See Chapter 6, p. 104 and Conclusion, p. 175 for further details on these warnings which, whether Amrita Pande likes it or not, have come true.

44 At the time of going to print, July 2017, the 2016 Bill has yet to be enacted by the Indian parliament. Meanwhile the exploitation of poor women continues in urban centres such as Hyderabad, as *Telangana Today* reports (Gopal, 19 June 2017), with government health inspectors demanding the urgent enactment of the Bill. While acknowledging the Bill's limitations, both Sheela Saravanan and Mohan Rao welcome the Indian government's prohibition of commercial surrogacy (2016).

Fertilisation and Embryology Authority (HFEA), this Bill would limit the practice of surrogacy in India to Indian infertile heterosexual married couples who can convince a relative to engage in so-called altruistic surrogacy.[45] Pande writes that

> ... what is critical for us is to view the surrogates as workers, and not as wombs, national resources or voiceless victims, so that they are the ones facilitating and participating in dialogues, and not just being discussed or being saved by an anxious patriarchal state (2016, p. 2).

Pande also makes the argument that "denying Indian women this particular *choice* (my emphasis), seems misplaced" (2016, p. 1). Elsewhere she suggests that such prohibitions will only result in surrogacy 'going underground' – the same old libertarian argument used in discussions regarding the introduction of the Nordic sex-buyer laws to eventually eliminate prostitution. She either does not know, or omits it from discussion, that in some Australian states that long ago legalised prostitution, the 'black market' was already four to five times the size of the legal industry in 2007 (Sullivan, 2007, p. 186). Similarly, it is well known that in

---

45 Indian supporters of 'altruistic' surrogacy have pointed out the Bill's discriminatory nature by banning Indian gay men as well as single people and de facto couples from using surrogacy. Since most foreigners have already been excluded from entering India for the purpose of surrogacy since 2015 by being unable to include a letter with their visa application from their country of residence stating that commercial surrogacy is legal (which of course it is not in most jurisdictions), the Indian government's 2016 bill is mostly for Indian citizens to debate. The largest group of foreigners still persisting with cheap surrogacy in India will be married heterosexual US citizens from the eight states (plus Washington DC) that have legalised surrogacy.

those eight US states where surrogacy is legal,[46] many people still opt for 'low cost surrogacy' in developing countries. Even if India or other poor countries legalised commercial surrogacy within a regulatory framework, the 'black market' would still happen. One thing that will stop it flourishing are *enforced* policies by countries from which the baby buyers hail, to make it a criminal offence to go overseas, procure a baby and bring it home (see Chapter 5, p. 83 and Conclusion, p. 157 for examples of such current laws in Australia, that are, however, not enforced). And of course educational campaigns that expose the exploitation of women and babies so that demand for surrogacy will shrink because it is deemed unethical – something that only 'unenlightened' people would want to engage in (see Conclusion, p. 177).[47]

Returning to the question of whether surrogacy would be ethical if it were defined as 'work' which, as Amrita Pande suggests, might enable womb mothers to negotiate better working conditions, higher pay and health protections and also use existing labour and occupational health policies to improve their workplace, I find it intriguing, that neither Pande nor other supporters of the 'surrogacy-as-work' ideology, attempt to *define* what the 'job' of growing and birthing a baby actually entails.

---

46 California, Connecticut, Delaware, Maine, New Hampshire, Nevada, Oregon and Rhode Island are the eight US states (plus Washington DC) that permit commercial surrogacy. For a list of surrogacy laws in US states, see <http://www.creativefamilyconnections.com/us-surrogacy-law-map>

47 Seventeen years after the sex buyer laws were introduced in Sweden in 1999, it is no longer seen as 'cool' for young men to buy prostituted women, but rather something that only 'losers' would do (Ekman, pers.com. 2014). Because of DNA matches, the sex buyer law has also sped up solving cold cases of murder, rape and organised crime.

If we stick just to the basics, the recruitment process to become a 'surrogate' begins with intrusive scrutiny of the woman's personal and social circumstances as to her suitability, and then informing her of the 'rules' to be followed over the next nine months (e.g. a strict diet and no sex with the husband). This is the prerequisite for medical tests including ultrasounds to establish her as a healthy baby carrier, followed by dozens of painful injections often with debilitating adverse effects to prepare her body for the embryo insertion. Next, if the embryo 'takes' and a pregnancy is established, follow days (sometimes months) of morning sickness (more drugs, more supplements). Question: do the surrogate 'workers' get a bonus at say, the end of the first trimester, if the baby has developed well? What about penalty rates for the 'job' on Saturdays, Sundays – after all it's 24/7 for nine months.[48] And what about holiday pay (except she can't take any holidays, not a single day). What is the remuneration scale for gaining adequate, but not too much, weight, for not having a miscarriage, for submitting to, and surviving, 'foetal reduction'? Closer to the birth, what if the baby upsets the pregnant woman's sleep, gives her gestational diabetes and makes her feel so constantly unwell that she gets depressed (more pills, more side effects)? What if she is one of those many pregnant women who develop pre-eclampsia, placenta praevia or even placental abruption towards the end of their pregnancy, all three life-threatening conditions for mother

---

48   The only other job I can think of that is 24/7 and can last for many months is that of an astronaut. But to my knowledge no astronaut has ever been asked to gestate and birth a baby while orbiting in space – and then give it away.

and child (increased when 'donor' eggs are used; see Chapter 2, p. 29) which need extended bed rest, sometimes for weeks? What will the occupation and health inspector have to say about these complications? How will they affect payment? Will she be paid more or less? Finally, most surrogacies end with a non-negotiable Caesarean section (and the baby is frequently pre-term) which is hard on the birth mother and needs extra time to recover from: surely the 'baby-worker' can rightfully expect a final bonus at this time.

The absurdity of trying to define the process of pregnancy and birth as 'work' should be patently obvious even from this incomplete description – as I have not mentioned any of the many different emotions that a pregnant 'surrogate' undergoes during the long nine months of her relationship with the developing child (homesickness for her own children; unannounced health inspections by her broker/pimp; sometimes daily questions/ skypes about the growing baby's condition from the anxious baby buyers). And what about thoughts that she will have to give away her baby that, just at this point in time, decides to get a hiccup and kick her in the tummy?

I suspect it is the impossibility of comprehensively listing the job description for 'surrogacy worker' that has made promoters of pregnancy and birth as a 'job' refrain from attempting to describe this complex process.

But there is another reason. Acknowledging that there is a *symbiotic* relationship between a pregnant woman and her developing baby, no matter whether she is a 'surrogate' or a 'real' mother – goes counter to the origin story of IVF and surrogacy which depicts 'making a baby' as a technological feat by 'technodocs' in which bits and pieces are combined – eggs, sperm, wombs, and of course the almighty genes. This origin story is far removed from the reality of a live woman's body that can grow a three-kilo-baby from an egg and a sperm cell. For potential baby buyers, thinking of a 'surrogate' as a petri dish eliminates the need for uncomfortable questions.

But no doubt I will be accused of being too 'literal', unable to understand the beneficial ramifications of surrogacy as 'labour' within the complex and misogynous global capitalist market, especially in a poor country.[49]

Again, I am reminded of parallels with prostitution. When prostitution survivors detail the extent of the violence, humiliation and abuse they experienced, they are shouted down by 'sex work' activists for being hysterical and weak, unable to enjoy the 'fun' sex buyers provide. They are admonished to enjoy the money and deal with the (few) negatives in a grown-up

---

49 I have noticed that proponents of surrogacy as labour draw on Maria Mies' important book *Patriarchy and Accumulation on a Word Scale* which was published in 1986. What Mies was referring to (similarly to Marilyn Waring in *Counting for Nothing: What Men Value and What Women are Worth*, 1988) was the exploitation and invisibility of women's (re)productive labour in the home, e.g. that it is never included in a country's GNP. It is intellectually dishonest (and in contravention of her 'moral right') to suggest that Mies would support the 'surrogacy-as-labour position'. As a founding member of FINRRAGE, Maria Mies has strongly critiqued reproductive technologies since the mid-80s, including surrogacy, as a form of capitalist commodification; see for example 'Why Do We Need All This? A Call Against Genetic Engineering and Reproductive Technology' (1985).

way: every job has downsides, right? (See prostitution survivors' accounts in Norma and Tankard Reist, 2016.)

Another argument used by supporters of the surrogacy-as-work mantra such as Sydney university academic Melinda Cooper, is to put it down "to squeamishness about intimate things becoming commercialised" when asked by a reporter why "we find it difficult to think of those who offer their bodies for surrogacy as workers" (Wade, 2017):

> It seems that when work becomes very bodily and intimate, people recoil, ... there's an element of moral disgust. When any kind of paid work touches on the body, or sexuality of family relations, such as surrogacy, people tend to want to sentimentalise and place it outside the category of labour ... we don't see offering our bodies for commercial extraction as dignified work.

I don't think that abolitionists are 'squeamish' about 'intimate things' such as the body and soul process of growing and birthing a child, and I reject that we are expected to 'sentimentalise' the process of rich buyers exploiting poor women's reproductive capacities within a capitalist marketplace. On the contrary, I suggest that we need to hear precisely what pro-work surrogacy supporters are telling us and object to it in the strongest possible terms:

For example, Amrita Pande provides us with an upsetting quote from one of the 'womb mothers' she interviewed (2015, p. 6):

> When I came here I told Doctor Madam that I am ready for all kinds of treatments – injections, medicines. I have suffered the pain and the bleeding. I almost got paralysis twice and had to be

hospitalized, because of side effects of some medicines. But I am not complaining about the pain. I worried, I cried and complained when my husband used to beat me up in front of my children. That pain is what you do not want. This kind of pain to the body I am willing to take – it will not be wasted – it will give me enough money to make me self-sufficient.

So did Amrita Pande take the woman to a health clinic, pay for a health check to make sure she was okay? Did she inform her (gently) that too many 'injections and medicines' can have disastrous consequences for women's health, often only surfacing many years later, so she should watch her health closely? Above all, did she pause to reflect what it means that abused women compare the pain from being beaten by a husband (which society condemns) with the pain experienced from a medical treatment that prepared her body for a pregnancy for someone else? Why should society not condemn this pain too? Might Pande not have decided that these adverse effects were proof of the inherent danger of surrogacy and started her campaign to stop it?

I do not know what her reaction was. But since that research, Pande has continued her worldwide crusade to establish that surrogacy is work and that "[T]he money earned through surrogacy often becomes a source of pride, and an indicator of their [women's] productivity" (2015, p. 6). This may well be so, but within an ethical framework that is based on striving for global human dignity and human rights that are based on a do-no-harm philosophy to your fellow human beings, surely the dangerous and exploitative nature of the surrogacy process is impossible to justify.

Another researcher, Sheela Saravanan who has also conducted ethnographic research with Indian 'surrogate mothers', contests Pande's emphasis that surrogacy is "work, an employment, a wage earning source, but more remunerative and hence a common option chosen by many women." She writes (Saravanan, 2018):

> This is a gross linguistic misinterpretation of the word *'kaam'* often used by surrogate mothers in India. When asked about their motivation they tend to say *'hum achha kaam kar rahe hain'*. A virtual translation of the word *kaam* is 'deed' as well as 'work', while what surrogate mothers mean by saying *'achha kaam'* is 'good deed' or a 'noble service', this has to do with their altruistic motivation rather than their reference to surrogacy as work. In the Indian cultural context, prostitution or infidelity is considered bad *'karma'* and this is what they are clarifying by saying that the IVF process does not include sleeping with anybody and also in the end gives a child to a couple and hence it is an 'achha kaam'. They are not saying that surrogacy should be a job option that all women should consider as a career, an employment that the government should promote for all women, nor are they saying that they would ever suggest this as an option for their daughters in the future.

And Saravanan continues:

> Surrogate mothers in my interviews say that 'I am doing this for my children. I am going through this agony so that my children have a better future, so that they can go to a good school, have a good education and need not do anything close to this in their lives and can manage to earn enough by doing other (just) kinds of work'.

It is crucial to understand that similarly to prostitution, in surrogacy we must not blame the women for being trapped in a dangerous situation. It is the *demand* for these 'services' that must be scrutinised and exposed. It is the global advertising campaigns that groom infertile couples and gay men that have led to the establishment of multibillion cross-border industries: money made literally from women's flesh.

Kumkum Sangari, author of *Solid:Liquid. A (trans)national reproductive formation* (2015) in which she continues her decades' long resistance to sex selection in India by now including surrogacy, assesses this mirage with steely irony (2015, p. 102):

> [In surrogacy] ... the propertyless woman turns by fiat into a propertied woman – an owner of ova and a uterus which can qualify as liquefiable or rentable assets. She is not really poor since she possesses potential capital – both her body and labour are a sign of entrepreneurial capacity and hidden capital.

And further, "At what class level will the labour time and risk of the surrogate be computed – that of corporate managers, doctors or clients, that of the low-waged informal service sector, or a 'standard' and thus arbitrary value? (2015, p. 82).

Questions such as these pinpoint the folly of trying to call surrogacy 'work'. Needless to say that a 'surrogate' or a prostituted woman will never receive full payment for their bodily assets and 'labour' as those profits go into the money bags of business entrepreneurs including middlemen. Delusions about earning good money that surrogacy supporters impart on women who are often destitute and living on the brink, remind me of assertions by American slave owners back in the 18th century that the quality of life slaves from Africa 'enjoyed' in their plantations was far superior to their prior down-trodden existence in Africa (Raymond, 2013, p. xxxiv).

These are pronouncements by the powerful who need the bodies (and souls) of the powerless so they can keep building cross-border empires and immorally amass wealth. They need to be resisted in the strongest possible terms (see Chapter 6).

To call surrogacy 'work' does not make it ethical.

There is another problem with the suggestion that surrogacy can be ethical. It is the unavoidable presence of eugenics during the pregnancy. Due to the increasing availability of new Non-Invasive Pre-natal Screening Tests (NIPTs) such as the IONA test developed by Premaitha Health from Manchester in the UK,[50] or Tranquility from Genoma in Switzerland, all pregnant women are increasingly subjected to tests that check for Down syndrome and other chromosomal abnormalities, but also for the sex of the developing baby. NIPTs can be done by the 10th week of pregnancy. The only 'solution' to one of these perceived gene mutations is abortion which, alarmingly, international meta-analyses confirm, is 'chosen' by 92.2% of women (see Achtelik, 2015, p. 58).

Women who have agreed to become 'surrogate' mothers have even less 'choice' in the matter: prospective baby buyers want a

---

50 Watch the promotional video for the IONA test and learn how "safe, fast and accurate" it is; <http://www.premaitha.com/the-iona-test> See also Melinda Tankard Reist's 2006 inspiring collection *Defiant Birth: Women Who Resist Medical Eugenics* for stories by women who continued their pregnancies despite alarming prenatal tests.

'perfect' child, hence already sperm and 'donated' or purchased egg cells are scrutinised for any genetic defects (and the sex where permitted). Often, after the embryo has been created by the fusion of sperm and egg, it is subjected to preimplantation genetic diagnosis (PGD) in which one cell is removed from the embryo and 'quality checked'. (The company Genoma lists over 80 monogenetic conditions, caused by one gene, that it can test for with PGD, <http://www.preimplantationgeneticdiagnosis. it/genetic-diseases-diagnosed-by-pgd.htm>). Only 'faultless' embryos are then inserted into the 'surrogate' mother's womb. But just to be sure, prenatal tests and repeated ultrasounds will still be requested and if an abortion is deemed necessary, the pregnant woman has to comply; the contract stipulates it. In my books this is called coercion – hence immediately disqualifying surrogacy as ethical.

Amrita Pande adds another disturbing dimension to this discussion. A quote from a participant in her research makes her voice her own, earlier quoted, disquiet that the practice of having babies for others may contribute to decades-long population control practices to prevent low-class women from having children in Asia and Africa. Pande calls this neo-eugenics and I agree.[51] Parvati, a 36-year-old Indian woman remembers when she went to the surrogacy clinic:

---

51 The FINRRAGE critique has always emphasised that reproductive technologies including surrogacy are only one side of the coin; the other is the merciless subjugation of poor 'undesirable' women wherever they are in the world through population control measures (e.g. sterilisation, long-term acting contraceptives and the DIY French abortion pill RU 486/

When I came here first time the doctor said I was too old to donate eggs but I could try for surrogacy. I underwent treatment – injections, vagina check. During one of these early checkups they realized that I was pregnant with my own child. We have just one child, and we have always wanted one more. But at that stage we needed the money more than a baby and I got my own baby aborted.

Having to abort your own baby so that you can avail yourself of the surrogacy 'work' to create another baby for strangers who can afford to pay for it, is surely one of the saddest stories I have heard. It exposes the callousness of the international surrogacy industry that uses women's poverty to impose their own rules. And it answers the question of this chapter: "can surrogacy be ethical?" with a resounding *No*.

In the next chapter I will discuss if regulation, be it of commercial or so-called altruistic surrogacy, could be the answer.

---

prostaglandin, see Klein *et al*. 1991, 2013). The Comilla Declaration (1989) elaborates on these points.

Chapter 5
Is regulation the answer?

The fundamental problem with focusing on regulation is that such an approach invariably precludes looking at the *roots* of the problem. In the case of attempting to 'regulate' surrogacy, this means that the very basic question of whether it could ever be justified to buy/rent a woman as a 'surrogate' and jeopardise the health of an egg 'donor', is not asked. Nor is the question asked whether *any one* should have the right to enter into a contract to buy and/or traffic a baby that is not yet conceived. It is also not clearly examined who the people are who are involved in these processes of exploitation. If it were, an examination would quickly show that they are well-to-do families, couples or individuals, straight or gay. They use the pain of their infertility or the inability to have their own genetic child to claim their *right* to buy (or at least solicit in so-called altruistic surrogacy) what they believe is their *entitlement*.

Regulatory frameworks exist within the confines of a neoliberal capitalist world view in which power differences between the social classes of women and men, as well as poor and rich people, lower and higher classes and different ethnicities are still firmly entrenched. As an example, it is well known that in the USA, a group of women who are targeted as 'surrogates' are low-income army wives. As US feminist critic Kathy Sloan puts it:

> Depending on the area of the country, it is estimated that between 20 and 50 percent of surrogates in the United States are military wives ... They are low-income (between $16,000 and $30,000 per year) and proven breeding stock, as they tend to get married and have their own children at very young ages ... While their husbands are serving their country abroad, they are told, they can 'serve' at home (Sloan, 24 April 2017).

Question: how do you 'regulate' the exploitation of a particular group of women so easily targeted? This question is of course even more pertinent in poor countries.

In a regulatory approach, a fundamental analysis that, in my view, inexorably leads to a *categoric* rejection of surrogacy, is pushed under the carpet and never even contemplated. Or, to put it differently: a regulatory inquiry does not start at the bottom and ask whether the practice of surrogacy should be abolished; it starts half way up and asks questions about how different aspects of surrogacy could or should be regulated. It is thus never a holistic search to understand the nature of the problem, but instead a *compartmentalised dissection* of the multiple problems arising from surrogacy. *Regulation enables the practice of surrogacy to continue. It institutionalises disconnection.*[52] (For more on this ur-patriarchal maxim, see Conclusion, p. 161).

---

52 In her brilliant book *Demon Lover. The Roots of Terrorism* (1989/2001), US author and international women's liberation activist, Robin Morgan said it succinctly: "If I had to name one quality as the genus of patriarchy, it would be compartmentalization, the capacity for institutionalizing disconnection" (p. 51).

The result is a complicated maze of legal recommendations that in the end make no one happy. People who want to see surrogacy abolished are dissatisfied. But so are prospective baby buyers, for whom these laws are far too restrictive. Again the regulation of prostitution should serve as a cautionary tale: whether it is in Germany, Holland or in a number of states in Australia, legalising prostitution has resulted in an illegal prostitution market which already in 2007 was four to five times the size of the legal industry (see Sullivan, 2007, p. 186). The only ones who profit from the long-winded processes devising regulatory frameworks are lawyers. And the IVF industry and their handmaidens: pro-surrogacy consumer groups who will always find a loophole to do what 'the clients want' (and pay for).

This is precisely what happened with a parliamentary inquiry in Australia into surrogacy in 2015/2016 (see below).

If one had any doubts about the power differentials involved in surrogacy, it is made clear through examining the economic status of the players. During the first decade of the 21st century, the practice of surrogacy in poor countries, especially in India, for rich baby buyers from around the world expanded significantly. What also expanded were critiques of the heartless exploitation of poor and low-class Indian women who were often kept in slave-like conditions in surrogacy houses for the whole duration of their pregnancy: exactly as had been predicted by Andrea Dworkin and Gena Corea in the 1980s (see Chapter 6, p. 104 and Conclusion, p. 175 for more details). Some good TV documentaries have been produced such as 'Google Baby' by Zippi Brand Frank (2009) and 'Made in India' by Rebecca Haimowiz and Vaishali Sinha (2010) who jarringly show the exploitation of poor women as 'surrogates'[53]

In Australia, the state of Victoria enacted new laws in 2010 that for the first time since 1995 allowed quite tightly regulated 'altruistic' surrogacy (see more in Chapter 6, p. 136). The discussion around surrogacy had been rekindled in 2006 when then Labor politician Stephen Conroy, a resident of Victoria, made headlines with his story that he and his wife, who had had a hysterectomy after ovarian cancer, were forced to travel to New South Wales to embark on an IVF surrogacy. They used two 'friends' as egg 'donor' and 'surrogate'. Sensing a great opportunity to fill his clinic's coffers, Dr John MacBain from Melbourne IVF launched an (unsuccessful) public plea to legalise commercial surrogacy in Australia (in Singer, 17 March 2009).

At the time of going to print, July 2017, commercial surrogacy remains prohibited in all seven states and territories.[54] In 2011,

---

53 In 'Google Baby', the Israeli 'entrepreneur' who introduces himself as the 'pregnancy producer'

provides customers with a cost effective solution using outsourcing of the surrogacy element to India as a way to lower prices. The preferred genetic material is selected by the clients from their computer: sperm and eggs are purchased on-line and multiple embryos are produced, frozen, packed and shipped by air to India – where they are implanted into the wombs of local surrogates. The customers arrive only at the end of the nine month pregnancy period to pick up their babies.

Long trailers for 'Google Baby' and 'Made in India' can be found on the Stop Surrogacy Now website under Resources <http://www.stopsurrogacynow.com/films/#sthash.PH66vVBS.dpbs>

54 Technically this is not quite correct. The Northern Territory has no laws on surrogacy. However, it also has no provisions for parentage orders.

the state of New South Wales followed Queensland and the Australian Capital Territory (ACT) in passing a law that makes it a criminal offence for citizens of these states to go abroad and embark on surrogacy arrangements. Unfortunately, to this day these laws have never been enforced. However, their introduction led to an increased activism by pro-surrogacy advocates, notable amongst them the aforementioned Sam Everingham, himself a baby buyer in India and in 2010 the founder of Surrogacy Australia and later Families through Surrogacy. As Everingham states clearly (see earlier, Chapter 4, pp. 47–48), the aim of pro-surrogacy groups is to introduce commercial surrogacy in Australia.

In December 2014, the cross-party House of Representatives Standing Committee on Social Policy and Legal Affairs announced it was holding a Round Table on the regulation and practice of surrogacy in Australia and international surrogacy arrangements in two separate sessions in February and March 2015.

To be fair to the Committee, they invited people from groups opposed to surrogacy such as Jo Fraser from ARMS (Association of Relinquishing Mothers), Penny Mackieson from VANISH (Victorian Adoption Network for Information and Self-Help), Sonia Allan, a long-time supporter of donor children, and myself as a representative of FINRRAGE. Nevertheless, at the meeting we found ourselves outnumbered by pro-surrogacy forces

---

In other words, the birth mother (and her partner if any) would remain the parents listed on the birth certificate. For these reasons, to my knowledge, no surrogacy has been attempted.

such as Sam Everingham from Surrogacy Australia/Families through Surrogacy, a prominent local IVF doctor, well known pro-surrogacy lawyer Stephen Page, an infertility counsellor praising surrogacy, and others. We also found out that unholy alliances had been made between some Committee members and pro-surrogacy groups who had already decided between themselves (and before the Round Table) that what should, and would, happen was an official parliamentary inquiry.[55]

And indeed this is what happened. On 2 December 2015, the House of Representatives Social Policy and Legal Affairs Committee called an 'Inquiry into the regulatory and legislative aspects of international and domestic surrogacy arrangements' and asked for Submissions to be sent to the Committee by early February 2016.

The Committee received 124 submissions, many of them written by people who put forward their individual cases stating that not having commercial surrogacy available in Australia deprived them of the 'right' to start their own families. It is disturbing to read how they cannot conceive of possible harms to 'surrogate' mothers, egg providers and the children born from such arrangements. They seem to have deep faith in Australia's lawmakers to regulate commercial surrogacy. Any problems, many of these individual submitters glibly suggest, could be overcome with 'counselling' (provided by the IVF industry, no

---

55 The one-sidedness of this process led me to send some 'Reflections on Roundtable' to all Committee members in which I spelt out some of the reasons why I hoped the Committee would adopt a more critical perspective on surrogacy rather than starting an Inquiry with the aim to regulate surrogacy (Klein 2015a).

doubt). Other submissions, amongst them many critical ones, were from legal academics, judges, relinquishing mothers, donor conceived groups, religious organisations and feminist groups, amongst them FINRRAGE and the Women's Bioethics Alliance.[56]

Due to a looming Federal Election on 2 July 2016, the Committee fast-tracked its work and managed to submit its Inquiry Report 'Surrogacy Matters' on 4 May 2016,[57] a day before the government went into caretaker mode. (If it had not done that, all their work might have been in vain.) The Government, through its Attorney General, is supposed to respond to the recommendations in any Inquiry Report within six months, but more than a year later, neither the Attorney General, nor any other government representatives, have responded. This delay is surprising, especially in the light of continued lobbying by pro-surrogacy groups and individuals, but also notwithstanding another surrogacy scandal in Cambodia (see Conclusion, pp. 158–159).

The 2016 Inquiry Report recommends that commercial surrogacy in Australia should remain illegal. Unfortunately, it also recommends that Australia needs best practice legislation on '*altruistic*' surrogacy in all its states and territories, in other words that the current surrogacy laws that vary from state to

---

56 The list of Submissions can be accessed at <http://www.aph.gov.au/ Parliamentary_Business/Committees/House/Social_Policy_and_Legal_ Affairs/Inquiry_into_surrogacy/Submissions>

57 The Inquiry Report 'Surrogacy Matters', 4 May 2017, can be accessed at <http://www.aph.gov.au/Parliamentary_Business/Committees/House/ Social_Policy_and_Legal_Affairs/Inquiry_into_surrogacy/Report>

state be replaced by a "nationally consistent legal framework." To achieve this aim, the Inquiry Report recommends that

> ... the Australian Government task the Australian Law Reform Commission with developing a model national law to regulate altruistic surrogacy, with particular consideration of four key principles – the best interests of the child, the surrogate's ability to make free and informed decisions, ensuring the surrogate is protected from exploitation, and legal clarity about the parent-child relationship (Inquiry Report, 2016, Foreword, p. v–vi).

The Law Reform Commission should be given twelve months to conduct an inquiry into the surrogacy laws of Australian States and Territories with a view to develop a model national law on 'altruistic' surrogacy. Within a further six months, the Attorney-General should request that the Council of Australian government (COAG) commit to consultation with all states and territories in relation to the proposed model and the overall desirability of having national uniform laws. The Inquiry Report suggests that the deliberations should not exceed twelve months (Inquiry Report, 2016, p. 20).

Those of us opposed to surrogacy were relieved to see that the Inquiry Report recommended keeping the prohibition of commercial surrogacy in Australia. But as most of us are also opposed to so-called altruistic surrogacy, we were not satisfied with the recommendation for the Law Reform Commission to develop a best practice national law on non-paid surrogacy. However, we were pleased that at least the Inquiry Report suggested a careful long-term framework to draft – and then discuss – these new laws state by state and territories. It would take two years before implementation could even begin. We saw this as a sign of hope that 'altruistic' surrogacy in Australia would not receive a boost from uniform laws anytime soon (which so far has been proven correct, both federally and in individual states/territories). Also, the various stages of drafting and considering a model national law on 'altruistic' surrogacy might enable groups opposed to surrogacy to have further input into these deliberations.

Unfortunately, however, as we had expected given the Terms of Reference that were published when the Government had called for submissions, the Committee had *not* considered whether the practice of surrogacy *per se* was morally, ethically and legally defensible. They had not gone to the root of the problem and asked fundamental questions. Instead, the 2016 Inquiry Report 'Surrogacy Matters' is a prime example of recommending a host of laws to *regulate* surrogacy, some of them so vague, that they would be, if ever implemented, easy to subvert. The Committee also missed a chance to ask whether the Australian government should initiate a *funded* national education campaign to encourage people *to stop* the practice of surrogacy. The Terms of Reference take for granted that surrogacy exists and cannot be stopped. Fifty years ago, many parliamentarians thought the same about smoking!

I include the Parliamentary Committee's Terms of Reference in full (below) because they show how easy it is to get embroiled in a host of big and small regulatory issues – compartmentalisation and disconnection at work – so that the big picture questions get pushed out of the frame. It is a 'not-seeing-the-wood-for-the-trees' problem; one that does not help us to stop a practice that is a human rights violation of women and children (Inquiry Report, 2016, p. ix). In fact, I contend that *attempts to regulate surrogacy act to legitimise it*.

But I also include the Terms of Reference because they will be very similar in any (western) country that decides to have a parliamentary inquiry into surrogacy with a view to regulate it.

Terms of reference

The House of Representatives Standing Committee on Social Policy and Legal Affairs will inquire and report into the regulatory and legislative aspects of international and domestic surrogacy arrangements, with a focus on:

- the role and responsibility of states and territories to regulate surrogacy, both international and domestic, and differences in existing legislative arrangements
- medical and welfare aspects for all parties involved, including regulatory requirements for intending parents and the role of health care providers, welfare services and other service providers
- issues arising regarding informed consent, exploitation, compensatory payments, rights and protections for all parties involved, including children
- relevant Commonwealth laws, policies and practices (including family law, immigration, citizenship, passports, child support and privacy) and improvements that could be made to enable the Commonwealth to respond approp-

riately to this issue (including consistency between laws where appropriate and desirable) to better protect children and others affected by such arrangements
- Australia's international obligations
- the adequacy of the information currently available to interested parties to surrogacy arrangements (including the child) on risks, rights and protections
- information sharing between the Commonwealth and states and territories, and
- the laws, policies and practices of other countries that impact upon international surrogacy.

It should be obvious that with Term of Reference such as these, all you will get are harms minimisation recommendations.

And that is exactly what happened. Ignoring the many submissions which suggested rejecting surrogacy *per se* as a human rights violation, the Committee's ten recommendations all remain within a regulatory framework.

For instance, on the question of 'adequacy of information on altruistic surrogacy', the recommendations suggest to develop a Government website

> ... to ensure it contains continually updated information on Commonwealth *support and service provision included that provided through medicare and the social security, welfare and child support mechanisms of the Commonwealth* (Inquiry Report, 2016, p. 21, my emphasis).

In other words, it looks like a given that the Commonwealth supports 'altruistic' surrogacy – no critical questions asked.

There are also glaring contradictions: The Committee appears not to notice that inquiring into 'Australia's international obligations', which include being a signatory to the UN Convention on the Rights of the Child, contradicts the next Term of Reference: 'the adequacy of the information currently available to interested parties to surrogacy arrangements (including the child) on risks, rights and protections'. The point is not whether the information on risks and protections available is correct or incorrect; the point is that under the UN Convention on the Rights of the Child, *surrogacy is not permitted*!

It is not that the Committee is unaware of these international obligations. On p. 28 of the Inquiry Report, they correctly list some of the treaties and agreements that Australia has signed. Amongst them are

> the Convention on the Rights of the Child; the International Covenant on Civil and Political Rights; the International Covenant on Economic, Social and Cultural Rights, and the Protocol to Prevent, Suppress and Punish Trafficking in Persons, Especially Women and Children, Supplementing the United Nations Convention against Transnational Organised Crime (Inquiry Report 2016, p. 28).[58]

---

58 Surprisingly, the Convention on the Elimination of All Forms of Discrimination Against Women (CEDAW) is missing from this list despite the fact that Australia is a signatory. See Chapter 6, pp. 150–151 for a Submission by an Italian NGO as part of the campaign Stop Surrogacy Now to the United Nations to address surrogacy within CEDAW.

But then, the Attorney-General's Department comments that "Australia's international human rights obligations only apply to people within its territory and subjects to its jurisdiction ..." (p. 29). In other words, they fail to see that currently occurring cases of so-called altruistic surrogacy in Australia *do already breach these international treaties*.

Furthermore, the Attorney-General's Department notes (p. 29):

> Consistent with the principle of State sovereignty, the relevant international human rights obligations in respect of individuals involved in surrogacy will generally be those of the State in which the relevant practice occurs.

Problem solved: not the Commonwealth's responsibility.

Nevertheless, the Committee is quite aware that intended baby buyers (aka 'commissioning parents') wilfully ignore laws in New South Wales, the Australian Capital Territory and Queensland which make it a criminal act to go overseas for surrogacy, and that breaking such laws has never resulted in a fine or jail term. The maximum jail terms applicable are two years, one year and three years respectively.

They refer to submissions from the Department of Immigration and Border Protection (DIBP) as well as the Department of Foreign Affairs (DFAT) which both declare that they are not able to take responsibility for identifying children born from surrogacy and that, "As such, there is effectively no Commonwealth Government regulation in relation to cases of offshore commercial surrogacy involving Australians" (p. 30). Nor does it appear that these two departments show a 'desire' "to manage the approximately 250 Australian families who enter into off shore commercial surrogacy arrangements, even when they do so in high-risk jurisdictions" (p. 32).

This means that as long as the sperm donor can prove paternity via a DNA test at an overseas Consulate or Embassy, 'his' child will be granted Australian citizenship and granted a passport. (However, some countries like the USA require the birth mother in a commercial surrogacy to be present when the baby is presented to Australian authorities.[59]) The Committee's wry comment on these revelations by DIBP and DFAT is that "this situation is far from ideal" (p. 32).

And so, in addition to their recommendation that the Attorney-General task the Australian Law Reform Commission with drafting a model national law for 'altruistic' surrogacy, the Inquiry Report also recommends that the Australian Government

> establish an interdepartmental taskforce (which should include eminent jurists with relevant expertise) to report in 12 months on ways to address the situation of Australians who choose [to] enter into offshore surrogacy arrangements ... (p. 33).

But amongst the issues it suggests this taskforce investigates, is the following: "considering whether it should be unlawful to engage in offshore surrogacy in any overseas jurisdiction where commercial surrogacy is prohibited" (p. 33).

---

59 Parentage issues are keenly investigated by an Expert's Group on Parentage/ Surrogacy at the Permanent Bureau of The Hague Conference on Private International Law, see pp. 88–91 of this chapter for further discussion.

It beggars belief that such a question should be 'considered.' Australians fully well know that breaching other countries' laws on, say, the importation of narcotic drugs, can lead to devastating consequences such as incarceration for life or even death sentences in the case of Indonesia.[60] And, since the 1994 Crimes (Child Sex Tourism) Amendment Act, Australian men caught when assaulting children sexually overseas, have been jailed (see Pearlman, 2017). And going overseas to Syria in order to fight as part of Daesh/ISIL means that such persons are not allowed to return to Australia.

Perhaps if jail or at least a big fine were foreshadowed to would-be seekers of off-shore surrogacy, it might stop them. Even more to the point, pro-surrogacy advocacy groups such as Families Through Surrogacy that hold annual conferences where they groom infertile and gay couples to engage in overseas surrogacy, should be *banned* (see my earlier comments in Chapter 4 on their 2014 conference, p. 47 and Conclusion, pp. 157–159). It is they (plus their 'sponsors' such as IVF clinics, egg brokers and overseas agents, and, very inappropriately, VARTA, the Victorian Assisted Reproductive Treatment Authority[61]) who

---

60 Schapelle Corby was jailed for twelve years for smuggling cannabis; <http://www.abc.net.au/news/2017-05-28/schapelle-corby-arrives-in-australia/8566052>. Convicted drug traffickers Andrew Chan and Myuran Sukumaran were executed by firing squad in Indonesia in 2015 despite pleas for clemency; <http://www.abc.net.au/news/2015-04-29/andrew-chan-and-myuran-sukumaran-executed/6426654>

61 The Victorian Assisted Reproductive Treatment Authority (VARTA) oversees the *Assisted Reproductive Technology Act 2008*. It is a taxpayer funded body and should therefore act as an objective, neutral body rather than

are unscrupulously encouraging people to have their own child at any price.[62] This is 'The Pimping of Surrogacy' (in analogy to Julie Bindel's 2017 book *The Pimping of Prostitution: Abolishing the Sex Work Myth*).

Returning to the 2016 Surrogacy Inquiry Report, on p. 31, the Committee notes

> the objections of submitters who oppose all forms of surrogacy on ethical grounds. However, given that there is no reasonable prospect of a worldwide ban on commercial surrogacy in the near future, the Committee must focus on how the potential risks and harms of international commercial surrogacy can be minimised.

It is nice to be acknowledged, but it is disheartening to see such a defeatist attitude which is particularly regrettable given the fact that some members of the Inquiry Committee do understand surrogacy's dangers for women and children. It is also wrong to not acknowledge that countries that allow commercial surrogacy are very few indeed: Georgia, Ukraine, Russia, Guatemala, some

---

co-organising, contributing to, and even acting as a sponsor for Families Through Surrogacy at their annual conferences.

62 Advertising for their June 2017 Melbourne Conference, Families Through Surrogacy promises to shed light on which states in Mexico still allow overseas surrogacies after surrogacy in the state of Tabasco was prohibited in 2015. We learn that 'Los Angeles Surrogacy' will recruit and screen Californian 'surrogates', but egg/sperm embryo creation happens in Cancun, as does the embryo transfer. The women then return to California for their pregnancy and birth. Another option is to go with 'Expecting Surrogacy' that recruits Mexican 'surrogates' with births also happening in California. And there is also 'Miracle Surrogacy', run by a Florida-based outfit where the entire process takes place in Mexico. The standard 'package' costs US$66,350 (advertising email from Families Through Surrogacy, 28 April 2017.)

states in Mexico and eight of the 52 states in the United States (plus Washington DC).[63]

We should thank the abolitionists of the 18th and 19th century that they continued to work fervently towards *abolishing* race slavery rather than just regulating it. Had they given in to harms minimisation solutions, race slavery might still be the norm in many countries. Initial efforts to curb slavery were based on regulating the slave trade which was seen as the evil rather than slavery itself, which was deemed "a state sanctioned 'economic sector'" (Raymond, 2013, p. iii) – a form of 'work' that brought major economic benefits to countries like Britain and the USA and could be made 'respectable' by cleaning up unsavoury work conditions. Similarly, surrogacy regulation is intent on providing fair and square 'working' conditions, so that abuses might be avoided, without acknowledging that *surrogacy itself is the abuse* which cannot be cleaned up and made to look 'nice' (see also my earlier comments in Chapter 4, pp. 52–66 on whether surrogacy should be called 'work').

Surrogacy abolitionists can also take heart from successful efforts to understand prostitution as violence against women and introduce laws that criminalise the sex buyers and pimps, but not the prostituted people (mostly women) in Sweden, Norway, Iceland, South Korea, France, Northern Ireland and Ireland, with other countries on their way to adopting what is

---

63 In Submission No. 17 to the Surrogacy Inquiry, Sonia Allan provides an excellent detailed overview of countries' laws (if any) on surrogacy; <http://www.aph.gov.au/Parliamentary_Business/Committees/House/Social_Policy_and_Legal_Affairs/Inquiry_into_surrogacy/Submissions>

called the 'Nordic Model' (see Meagan Tyler's summary of sex buyer laws in Norma and Tankard Reist, eds. 2016, pp. 213–225). It is crucially important that we compare debates on 'free and forced' 'sex work' with 'well regulated surrogacy' in, say, the USA, and supposedly substandard practices in poor and developing countries. Under close scrutiny, these differences crumble: at the end of the day, it is always the (poorer) woman who hands over her 'home made' baby to (richer) baby buyers, and it is the baby who is deprived of her or his birth mother. And when a court case ensues, it is highly unlikely that the 'surrogate' and her family have the financial means to fight for, for example, unpaid medical expenses or custody of her child(ren).

To repeat: it is time to seriously consider criminalising baby buyers and their 'pimps' who give oxygen to this dehumanising trade in women and babies and profit from it. It is equally important *not* to criminalise so-called surrogate mothers and egg providers.

It also needs to be pointed out that not all Parliamentary Reports end with recommendations for regulating surrogacy. In February 2016, the Swedish Parliament published its report *Olika vägar till föräldraskap* (Different Paths to Parenting) recommending that altruistic surrogacy should join the existing prohibition of commercial surrogacy in Sweden (see Swedish Government, 2016, English Summary).[64]

---

64 On 19 June 2016, the Stockholm UN Association supported all of the recommendations in *Olika vägar till föräldraskap* and joined Rosberg and her parliamentary committee in demanding the prohibition of all types of

The author of the Parliamentary Report, Justice Eva Wendel Rosberg, says there were two main concerns: Firstly, there was no research on how people born from surrogacy feel about their origins. Secondly, Rosberg and colleagues felt that it was impossible to say that the 'surrogate' mother has made a truly uncoerced decision. Rosberg emphasised that these concerns pertained to both commercial and 'altruistic' surrogacy: "Even those who carry babies for relatives, she said, may be pressured by family expectations" (in *The Economist*, 13 May 2017). The report also suggested that Swedes should be discouraged from going overseas for surrogacy by making public the legal problems that will make it impossible for them to bring children from surrogacy back to Sweden. Australia should take a leaf out of the Swedish report.

Ever the optimists, the FINRRAGE Summary of Principles on Surrogacy in their Submission to the 2016 Surrogacy Inquiry Commission (p. 6) ended with the words: "FINRRAGE believes a world without surrogacy is possible."[65]

And indeed we do. But we also know that the road to this end will be hard and plastered with many obstacles. One of these is the ongoing labour of the Permanent Bureau of the Hague Conference on Private International Law, started in 2011,

---

surrogacy in Sweden (<http://www.stopsurrogacynow.com/updates-from-sweden-and-minnesota-usa/#sthash.VoF4LVCb.dpbs>). However, at the time of finishing this book, July 2017, the Swedish Government has still not voted on this report (Ekman, pers. com, July 2017).

65 The FINRRAGE Submission No. 70 can be viewed here: <http://www.aph.gov.au/Parliamentary_Business/Committees/House/Social_Policy_and_Legal_Affairs/Inquiry_into_surrogacy/Submissions>

intending to draft an international convention on cross-border surrogacy similar to the existing convention on intercountry adoption. However, such an international convention would need the approval of all 77 member states, as well as all members of the European Union to legalise surrogacy which, of course, hardly any country currently does! It is thus fair to say that such a surrogacy convention is years, if not decades away. It may never eventuate, given the very different laws – and views – these countries have on surrogacy which would have to be brought in line (see also below, pp. 99–102 below for a much better suggestion which is an international convention *to abolish* surrogacy).

Faced with these logistical hurdles, it appears that since 2015, the 'Parentage/Surrogacy Project' has become the focus of the Hague Conference that they seem to think might be most realistic to achieve. So their project to 'regulate' surrogacy internationally has not been abandoned; they continue to legitimise it.

Still, it is interesting that 'legal parentage or filiation' is the chosen emphasis. Even within a regulatory framework, one would think that other aspects of surrogacy such as the health of so-called surrogate mothers and egg providers, or the human rights of the children born through surrogacy would rank equally with 'parentage'. But no, it is the interests of the baby buyers – and specifically the sperm donors – that are given priority. Are we surprised?

Long-time critic of reproductive technologies including surrogacy, US Professor of Women's Studies and Medical Ethics, and FINRRAGE co-founder, Janice Raymond, was already predicting the focus on parentage in 1993 when she said to

PhD candidate, Australian Kathy Munro, in an interview (Munro, 1997, p. 64):

> If women are different to men, as in pregnancy, then what they get, men have to have access to that too. So that you can't define motherhood on a standard that is basically pertinent to womanhood, you have to define parenthood on a standard that is very much related to male parenthood, so it's genetics, and pregnancy doesn't count. Pregnancy doesn't count because men can't do it. So what do they base the standard of parenthood on? What men can do. What can they do? They can contribute genes.

And it is indeed these male genes that are the crux of the patriarchal concepts of 'gestational pregnancy' and 'parentage'.

In 2015, the Attorney-General nominated Chief Justice John Pascoe of the Federal Circuit Court of Australia as its delegate on the Experts' Group on Parentage. Justice Pascoe is a respected judge who does understand the harms of surrogacy to women and children. The first meeting of the Experts' Group was convened from 15 to 18 February 2016. As the Conclusion in the Meeting Report stated, unsurprisingly:

> The Group determined that, owing to the complexity of the subject and the diversity of approaches by States to these matters, definitive conclusions could not be reached at the meeting as to the feasibility of a possible work product in this area and its type or scope.

Nevertheless, not one to give up, the Experts' Group recommended that their mandate should continue and tasked the Permanent Bureau "to undertake the necessary work with a view to preparing a next meeting of the Group and allocate resources accordingly" (Hague Conference on Private International Law,

'Report of the February 2016 meeting of the experts' group on parentage/surrogacy', p. x).

Kathy Sloan, a US author, activist and original signatory to the campaign Stop Surrogacy Now who is tirelessly exposing the patriarcho-capitalist machinations of the surrogacy industry in the USA, adds an important insight to the Experts' Meeting in the Hague. Shortly before their meeting in February 2016, the leader of the US delegation to the Experts' Meeting, US State Department Employee, Lisa Vogel, convened a meeting of US surrogacy industry representatives – prominent surrogacy attorneys and owners of surrogacy agencies with whom she was clearly well acquainted – to canvass their opinions on "how to make the case to other countries for an international surrogacy enabling agreement based on the US 'exceptionalist' model of surrogacy in all its forms" (Sloan, 24 April 2017).[66]

Sloan, who participated in this meeting via phone, continues: "The main priority of the industry and its US government partner is determining the best way to ensure enforceable contracts and establishing citizenship for the children in the buyers' home country." And she adds: "In sum, [the meeting] was like an industry convention with the US government there to serve its interests."

The 2017 Experts' Meeting in the Hague on parentage/surrogacy on 31 January to 3 February went one step further than

---

66 The myth of the supposedly 'exceptionally' well-regulated surrogacy industry in the USA will be discussed in Chapter 6, pp. 148–149. Interesting for Australian readers is Kathy Sloan's comment that "A vocal non-US participant was Australia's most prominent surrogacy attorney Stephen Page" (Sloan, 24 April 2017).

the 2016 gathering: "The majority of the Group expressed the view that the recognition, by operation of law, of foreign judicial decisions on legal parentage in a multilateral instrument *would be feasible*" (Hague Conference on Private International Law, 'Report of the February 2017 meeting of the experts' group on parentage/surrogacy', p. 2, my emphasis).

And further:

> Noting that legal parentage, particularly in the context of ISAs [International Surrogacy Arrangements], was a complex and evolving topic, the Group emphasized the importance of concentrating on the PIL [Private International Law] aspects, and on the need for practical solutions, with *one of the key aims being to secure continuity in the parent-child legal status* (as above, p. 3, my emphasis).

Put differently, of all the troublesome aspects of international surrogacy, it is *Fathers' Rights* that appear to be advancing: Aristotle 2.0 (see Chapter 2, pp. 27–28 and Chapter 6, p. 137). Plus ça change, plus c'est la même chose!

If member states of the Hague Conference on Private International Law (HCCH) eventually were to go further and, despite the obstacles, decided to embark on a broad based international convention on cross-border surrogacy, this would pose serious problems for women's and human rights activists. It would be regulation on a grand scale and would force countries that currently prohibit surrogacy (the overwhelming majority of all countries) to change their national laws.[67]

---

67 But there are always ways and means to find loopholes that benefit the baby buyers. On 18 Dec 2016, Stephen Page had exciting news:

When I came across the information that, already in 2014, The International Institute of Social Studies (ISS) of Erasmus University Rotterdam in The Hague had convened an 'International Forum on Intercontinental Adoption and Global Surrogacy' (11–13 August 2014), I thought this was good news; obviously other people must have been worried about such a potentially wide-ranging convention on surrogacy which would cement it as internationally recognised.

The report from the Thematic Area 5, 'Global Surrogacy Practices', described the event as "a landmark conference that brought together nearly a hundred scholars, women's health and

---

> In a groundbreaking decision, for the first time ever, the Family Court of Australia has registered a US surrogacy order. The effect of the Australian order means, that for all purposes the US order can be enforced in Australia and that the parents of the child as recognised by the US order are recognised as the parents of the child in Australia.

Page further explains that some US states issue pre-birth parentage orders which name the 'baby buyers' as the parents rather than the 'surrogate' mother. And:

> This means, for example, that the only people who have been granted parental responsibility for the child, in effect for the *Australian Passports Act*, are the parents, not the surrogate. *Therefore the surrogate's consent for new Australian passports for the child will not be required* (my emphasis).

This is 'excellent' news as it gets the birth mother out of the way and, with her, any potentially unwelcome scenes at the Australian Consulate/ Embassy. However, Page cautions that pre-parentage orders can only be issued for 'altruistic' surrogacies, and the IPs (intended parents) must exert great caution and, *always*, get legal advice. No doubt this new loophole will be exploited by pro-surrogacy advocates; <http:// surrogacyandadoption.blogspot.com.au/search?updated-max= 2017-01-29T15:34:00%2B10:00&max-results=7&start=21&by-date=false>

human rights advocates and policymakers from 27 countries"
(Darnovsky and Beeson, 2014).

Unfortunately, however, the Abstract of 'Global Surrogacy
Practices' reveals that most participants appear to have envisaged
a *regulatory* approach in their deliberations of surrogacy. And
again "resolving the legal and citizenship status of children"–
in other words parentage issues yet again – is emphasised.
Furthermore, and very contentious, the Abstract foreshadows
the language of 'surrogacy-as-work' that is then employed
throughout the report – without any proper discussion whether
the 24/7 gestation of new life from a woman's own body could
ever be defined as 'work' (see my earlier discussion of surrogacy
as 'work,' Chapter 4, pp. 52–66). As Darnosvky and Beeson write
(2014, p. x):

> Participants affirmed the importance of resolving the legal and
> citizenship status of children resulting from international surrogacy
> arrangements. In addition, they highlighted the need for greater
> policy and public attention to a wide range of effects on all the
> parties involved, particularly *women working as surrogates* and the
> children they gestate and bear (my emphasis).

Who exactly were the invited delegates to this Forum? As it turns
out, only 24 people were listed by name at the end of the report
as attendees in Thematic Area 5 'Global Surrogacy Practices';
the rest of the 'close to one hundred' participants whose main
interest appears not to have been surrogacy, but intercountry
adoption, remain (with very few exceptions) nameless. Of those
24 people listed, more than half are well known *liberal* feminists
who favour regulation and reject the abolition of surrogacy –
including the writers of the report, US feminists Marcy Darnovsky

and Diane Beeson. This explains the overwhelming focus on regulation in 'Global Surrogacy Practices'.

Nevertheless, there appear to have been some other delegates present – possibly in the two joint sessions with the Intercountry Adoption Thematic Area – who spoke out against surrogacy as a human rights violation and violence against women and wanted it banned. In the section 'Regulation vs. Prohibition: Mutually Exclusive Alternatives'? Darnovsky and Beeson write (2014, p. 36):

> Participants were divided about whether intercountry commercial surrogacy should be more effectively regulated, or prohibited altogether. Some held a strong position; some were uncertain. Many were open to the possibility that an international convention could mitigate many of the problematic practices and consequences associated with intercountry surrogacy.
>
> Some Forum participants, however, questioned whether an international convention might wind up undermining the prohibitions on commercial surrogacy that many jurisdictions have put in place, often on the grounds that the practice violates the human dignity of both the child and the gestational mother. From this point of view, there was concern that an international convention might normalise commercial surrogacy, and/or fail to significantly reduce the human rights violations it entails. Questions were also raised about whether intercountry surrogacy might, at least in some circumstances, constitute baby selling, or violate the Convention on the Rights of the Child by failing to preserve his or her identity, nationality and family relations.

Indeed! However, such more radical views were clearly side-lined and not further discussed. As Darnovsky and Beeson state (2014, p. 37):

> Other participants, whatever their assessment of the potential likelihood and efficacy of an international convention, supported regulation of commercial surrogacy rather than prohibition for reasons based in pragmatism, principle or both. Some argued for regulation as the most effective way to provide urgently needed protections for the women and children involved in commercial surrogacy arrangements. Others pointed out that bans on commercial surrogacy would be politically very difficult to enact in many of the jurisdictions in which it is currently established practice, and that regimes permitting altruistic but not commercial surrogacy arrangements would be difficult to oversee.

The last point is particularly puzzling. Why would it be "difficult to oversee" paid surrogacy in countries that allow so-called altruistic surrogacies? To put it bluntly, if commercial surrogacy is legally prohibited in a country, breaking such a law constitutes a crime. This is the case currently in Australia. It is not difficult to regulate. An analogy would be to argue that smoking in public places can't be banned, because people are allowed to smoke in the privacy of their own home. Australia *has* banned smoking in public places.

Darnovsky and Beeson continue (2014, pp. 37–38, my emphasis):

> Some base their support for permitting effectively regulated commercial surrogacy on principled arguments about women's agency, and point to evidence that many women *working* as surrogates are grateful for the opportunity to earn a significant

amount of money. They simply want better *working* conditions and protections against health risks, as well as a reduction in stigma associated with such arrangements.

I have already discussed the deeply problematic nature of calling surrogacy 'work' (see Chapter 4, pp. 52–66), but it is illuminating to read how the notion that surrogacy constitutes 'work' slips effortlessly from the pen of these two liberal US feminist writers and pervades the whole report. They also appear to either wear rose-tinted glasses, or wishing to knowingly blur the real difference between abolitionists and regulators. As they state (2014, p. 37):

> Despite the tendency of some to consider 'prohibition' and 'regulation' of commercial surrogacy as opposed and non-overlapping positions, it is possible to envision a wide range of legal or policy approaches that might effectively minimise or eliminate the problematic aspects of intercountry surrogacy. These could include criminal or civil sanctions against intermediaries but not other parties involved with surrogacy arrangements; a variety of rules about legal parentage of resulting children and preservation of records; requirements about the content, timing and enforceability of surrogacy contracts; requirements about the status and/or conduct of intermediaries; rules prohibiting discrimination against commissioning parents or surrogates on the grounds of marital status, sexual orientation, and disability; enforceable protections for the health and safety of surrogates; screening requirements for commissioning parents, etc. There might also be laws to restrict commercial arrangements to people domiciled within the countries that accept them, and/or to limit transnational arrangements to situations in which both countries agree to recognise legal parentage and citizenship of any resulting child.

What this last quote shows is a list of *regulatory harms minimisation measures*. This is not prohibition. Prohibition means no surrogacy is permitted. Why is 'no-means-no' so difficult to understand?

I have quoted extensively from this report because it shows the sink hole that is regulation. The critical issue that goes to the root of the problem of whether surrogacy should exist at all, whether it is a moral and ethical undertaking for so-called 'intended parents' (baby buyers) to ask 'surrogate' mothers and egg 'donors' to risk their lives and create children that have never asked to be separated from their birth mothers, is not properly discussed. Instead, the discussion defaults to secondary regulatory issues which may be important in a harms minimisation context, but are worlds apart from the existential questions that surrogacy poses: why some people – wealthy individuals – believe they have the *right* to expect poorer people – and exclusively females – to grow and deliver them babies, whether for love or money.

If these were not enough reasons to reject regulation and harms minimisation policies, there is also the fact that they create a behemoth of unruly laws and a postmodern heaven of neoliberal fantasies of freedom and 'choice' for some.

Importantly, these regulations only wait to be scratched at the surface so that weak spots can be found and exploited. Welcome to a black surrogacy market enabled by regulation!

To sum up this chapter on whether regulation is the answer, a more mundane reason why many people favour regulation and harms minimisation instead of prohibition, is uneasiness and fear: the widespread *fear of saying 'No' to someone*, especially when babies are concerned. I am reminded of a tea break at a pro-surrogacy conference in 2014 when I started to have a good conversation with an unknown woman about the dangers to women and children from surrogacy. She agreed with me – but then said, as the bell rang to call us back to our seats, "but those poor gay men who so desperately want their own babies, we can't really say no to them." It is this nervousness and fear of hurting others' feelings – and appearing to be homophobic in this case – that is so pervasive in our society – especially among women. It often stops us from having a really good look at fundamental problems with a number of social justice issues. And then bravely saying *No*.

Fortunately for critics of surrogacy, on 23 March 2015, a group of mostly European feminist abolitionists (but including the US Center for Bioethics and Culture that hosts Stop Surrogacy Now) was brave – and angry – enough to issue a challenge to the Hague Conference on Private International Law (HCCH). They commented on The Hague's Preliminary Documents No 3 B of March 2014 and No 3 A of March 2015, accusing the HCCH of hiding its attempts to draft an international pro-surrogacy convention from public scrutiny since 2011 and only relying on surrogacy proponents (p. 6):

> The Permanent Bureau only included the perspectives of professionals who are actively involved in surrogacy, not only stakeholders but promoters of the practice.
>
> The opinion of these professionals has the potential to facilitate the mutual recognition of filiation through surrogacy, thereby supporting their activities in this domain.

The question of any potential ban against the practice was not even raised, despite the fact that it is strictly forbidden in a number of countries.

The inspiring proposal outlines the need for an *'International Convention for the Abolition of Surrogacy,'* which, the authors suggest, be modelled on the "1926 Slavery Convention and the Supplementary Convention on the Abolition of Slavery, the Slave Trade, and Institutions and Practices Similar to Slavery in 1956" (p. 23).

In their document, the French Collectif pour le Respect de la Personne (CoRP), Cadac (Coordination des associations pour le droit à l'avortement et à la contraception), CLF (Coordination lesbienne en France), La Lune (association of lesbian feminists), the European Women's Lobby, the Center for Bioethics and Culture (USA), the Swedish Women's Lobby and several other associations and individuals (Gertrud Årström, Sweden; Kajsa Ekis Ekman, Sweden; Elfriede Hammerl, Austria; and Alice Schwarzer, Germany) set out their reasons why we need an International Convention for the Abolition of Surrogacy instead of any regulatory instruments (CoRP *et al.* 2015), many of them very similar to what I have discussed in this book.[68]

The feminist authors emphasise that surrogacy is a practice of exploitation that contravenes existing International Human Rights Conventions and list them (2015, pp. 17–22):

---

68 This important document needs to be distributed as widely as possible and further developed by the original authors and others. An English version is available at <https://collectifcorp.files.wordpress.com/2015/01/surrogacy_hcch_feminists_english.pdf>

- The Convention on Intercountry Adoption;
- The United States Slavery Convention;
- The International Convention on the Rights of the Child;
- The Optional Protocol to the Convention of the Child on the sale of children, child prostitution and child pornography;
- The Protocol to Prevent, Suppress and Punish Trafficking in Persons, Especially Women and Children, supplementing the United Nations;
- The Convention against Transnational Organized Crime;
- Regional Instruments (such as the Orviedo Convention which stipulates 'The human body and its parts shall not, as such, give rise to financial gains.'[69]

And they summarise their argument succinctly: "Any instrument tending to organize or regulate the practice of surrogate motherhood is inconsistent with the international texts currently in force" (p. 13). This includes the existing Convention on Intercountry Adoption (p. 17):

> The Hague Conference cannot simultaneously combat the marketing of children and the exploitation of the reproductive capacities of others in the context of international adoption and, on the other hand, organize the same practices in the context of surrogacy, provided that safeguards (weak ones, moreover) are created.

Of the International Convention of the Rights of the Child, they say (pp. 17–18):

> Surrogacy violates Article 7 § 1 of the Convention on the Rights of the Child.

---

69 This is, of course, precisely what happens with IVF clinics, brokers, pro-surrogacy advocacy groups – the pimps of surrogacy – who profit hugely from the bodies of the so-called surrogate and egg 'donors'.

Article 35 of The International Convention on the Rights of the Child stipulates 'State Parties shall take all appropriate national, bilateral and multilateral measures to prevent the abduction of, or traffic in children for any purpose or in any form' ... [Surrogacy] represents the sale of a child in the sense of Article 35 of the International Convention on the Rights of the Child.

They conclude their proposal for an International Convention for the Abolition of Surrogacy (situated within the United Nations framework for conventions) with the following words (p. 23):

In order to render a ban on surrogacy and the struggle against this practice fully effective, provisions also need to be established stipulating legal punishments that criminalize surrogacy, or at least the intermediary activities surrounding surrogacy.

These stipulations could either constitute part of the abolition convention or be included in an additional protocol thereto. This second option could enable the abolition convention to generate broader support concentrated on banning the principle and measures to be taken to cause the practice to decrease. This would permit the most willing States to establish criminal cooperation to more effectively combat the practice.

This protocol could be inspired by texts related to criminal cooperation that already exist relative to the field of trafficking in its broader sense, including:

- The Convention for the Suppression of the Traffic in Persons and of the Exploitation of the Prostitution of Others;
- The Protocol to Prevent, Suppress and Punish Trafficking in Persons, Especially Women and Children, supplementing the United Nations Convention against Transnational Organized Crime;

- The Optional Protocol to the Convention on the Rights of the Child on the sale of children, child prostitution and child pornography.

The idea of an International Convention for the Abolition of Surrogacy is a really exciting development. It gives me tremendous hope to know that there are feminists around the world – individuals and groups – with whom we can continue to work jointly to defend women's und children's human rights and dignity against the violation that is surrogacy.[70]

In the next chapter I will present an overview of past and current feminist resistance to surrogacy.

---

70 The authors of the International Convention for the Abolition of Surrogacy addressed their document to the Hague Conference on Private International Law (HCCH), asking for it to be distributed to all members and wanting to be included in further discussions. It appears the HCCH did not do either. I can find nothing on their website relating to this proposal despite them listing a January 2016 'Background Note for the Meeting of the Experts' Group on the Parentage/Surrogacy Project; <https://assets.hcch.net/docs/8767f910-ae25-4564-a67c-7f2a002fb5c0.pdf> The International Convention for the Abolition of Surrogacy would have been a perfect fit for this Background Note.

Chapter 6
Resistance – past and present

Today's radical resistance to surrogacy by feminists, human rights activists and other concerned groups who are coming together in the international campaign Stop Surrogacy Now (see below, pp. 145–153) is by no means a new phenomenon. Resistance started in the early 1980s when surrogacy was thrown into the spotlight in the USA after entrepreneurs such as Noel Keane in Michigan had opened surrogate agencies in the late 1970s. Keane saw himself as a pioneer and champion in a movement of 'breeder women' (Gena Corea's term) that saw the establishment of close to twenty surrogate agencies all over the USA by the mid-1980s (in Corea, 1985, pp. 213–14).

It is interesting to note that all the same issues that are discussed today were aired more than 30 years ago: Should surrogacy only be available for heterosexual couples, or should single and gay men be allowed to hire a 'surrogate'? Should surrogacy only be 'altruistic', or should it have to be paid for? And which women are to be 'surrogates': poor women who need the money to survive, or any 'special' woman with a big heart who is keen to fill the empty arms of suffering infertile couples? Is surrogacy a benevolent service, or is it exploitation? Keane created an 'educational video' to be shown in high schools called 'Special Ladies' to "... pimp young women into surrogacy using the appeal of altruism as a seasoning process – a gentle strategy of procurement casting surrogacy as a supreme act of female giving" (in Raymond, 1993/1995, p. 44). And what about the possibility of sex selection? The requirement for a 'surrogate' to undergo prenatal testing followed by abortion, if the product child is deemed 'not perfect'?

These are social justice issues of poverty, class, race, sex and disability.

Feminist criticism was quick at hand. Among the first was the brilliant writer Andrea Dworkin who, already in 1983, predicted the exploitative 'farming' of 'surrogates' in stables, preferably in poor countries – as we have seen since in India, Thailand, Cambodia, Nepal, Ukraine and Mexico.

Calling surrogacy 'reproductive prostitution' in analogy to sexual prostitution taking place in brothels, Dworkin compared the brothel model to the farming model (1983, p. 174):

> The farming model relates to motherhood, women as a class planted with the male seed and harvested; women used for the fruit they bear, like trees; women who run the gamut from prized cows to mangy dogs, from highbred horses to sad beasts of burden.

Similar concerns emerged in a spate of feminist books on reproductive technologies that were published in the 1980s. The first international anthology was *Test-Tube Women: What Future for Motherhood* (Arditti, Duelli Klein and Minden, 1984/1989),[71]

---

71 *The Custom-Made Child: Women-Centered Perspectives*, edited by Helen B Holmes, Betty Hoskins, and Michael Gross was published in 1981. It was the Proceedings of the 1979 workshop 'Ethical Issues in Human Reproduction

in which 33 writers asked urgent questions about the impact on women from the quickly unfolding brave new world of test-tube babies. (Louise Brown had only been born in 1978.) The book also explored the other side of the coin: dangerous sterilisation and contraceptive technologies often enforced on poor women in the west and in the so-called third world as population control.[72]

Amongst the contributors to *Test–Tube Women* was US journalist Susan Ince with her first-hand account of answering a newspaper advertisement from a 'reputable' surrogacy agency 'Inside the Surrogate Industry' (pp. 99–116). As Ince completes the application process – she does get accepted as a 'surrogate' – she is shocked by the lack of medical and psychological safeguards as well as the extensive control over a 'surrogate's' life by the company. This includes the way surrogacy is presented

---

Technology, Analysis by Women' in Amherst, MA, USA. Canvassing a wide range of issues from prenatal diagnosis and sex preselection to the ethics of manipulations of reproductive technologies, the book heralded the arrival of great concern about these new technologies for feminists that came to dominate the 1980s until the late 1990s.

72 The tone of the book is one of great urgency and alarm. Although IVF and related technologies had only just begun to be developed, crucial issues such as dangers for women from drugs and operations, eugenics, prenatal testing sex selection, the very question of existence for disabled people, and the development of the artificial womb were all canvassed. Re-reading it in 2017 is upsetting because the prescience of these writings, that are by and large no longer discussed today, is impressive. Many foreshadowed technological developments have indeed become mainstream, but the 'bigger picture' about the control of patriarchal institutions over women's reproductive lives and motherhood – the 'Background' – is hardly discussed any more. It needs urgent revisiting (see Conclusion, p. 160).

to the world: "Even the glowing descriptions of the surrogates sound remarkably like a happy hooker with a heart of gold" (p. 115). Reflecting on her own experience she warns that, "... we must not participate in a quiet liberal complicity with the new reproductive prostitution. It is our challenge to pay attention to our feminist visionaries, and to expose the surrogate industry during its formation" (p. 115).

Test-Tube Women was followed by Gena Corea's outstanding work: *The Mother Machine: Reproductive Technologies from Artificial Insemination to Artificial Wombs* (1985). Corea's words were a clarion call to women to look behind the 'Foreground' of reproductive technologies, as they are sold to us as a benign 'cure' to ease infertile women's pain, to the 'Background': the very real possibility that in the future, medical control over 'ordinary' women of childbearing age will amount to patriarchal control over who in the world is allowed to have children and determine their 'quality' (see Conclusion, pp. 168–169).

And indeed, the rapid proliferation of finding more and more so-called (genetic) diseases and 'abnormalities' via prenatal testing has led to a gradual expansion of IVF clinics' customers way past people with a fertility issue (e.g. by deciding to use IVF and preimplantation genetic diagnosis, PGD, to ensure the embryo is disease free).

Corea also devotes a whole chapter to 'Surrogate Mother-hood: Happy Breeder Woman' (pp. 213–249) which, in the early 1980s, was always of the 'traditional' kind: the hired woman was inseminated with the sperm of the intended father; aka baby buyer. This practice changed in the mid-1980s when the embryo transfer method was perfected and IVF doctors created the myth of the 'gestational carrier' who supposedly has no attachment to the growing baby because the embryo implanted in her womb does not contain any of her genes. (see below, p. 133). This myth survives to this day and is one of the mainstays of the surrogacy industry, unfortunately believed by so-called surrogates all over the world who maintain they have no connection with their developing child.

The radical feminist quest to find out more about these technologies and shed light on what 'gifts' benevolent (male) scientists and doctors were ready to bestow on women worldwide, continued with an international panel at the 2nd International Interdisciplinary Congress on Women, in Groningen, Holland, in April 1984. Ominously entitled 'Death of the Female?,[73] at the end of the presentations on the future of reproductive technologies for women, the 500 participants urgently demanded the foundation of an international network to counteract what was beginning to look increasingly like

---

73 The conference proceedings were published as *Man-Made Women* in 1986/1987 (Corea *et al.*). Again the papers show the urgency with which feminists approached these technologies: not simply as the latest technological feat (or failure), but as a systematic new framework of an international medical take-over of women's reproductive lives. As Janice Raymond cautions us in her Preface (1986/1987, p. 13):

This does not mean that the anti-feminism of the 'technodocs' and their reproductive engineering proposals are always intentional, planned or conspiratorial. It was Hannah Arendt who gave us the concept of the 'banality of evil' ... Many 'technodocs' do not harm women because they are ontologically evil, monstrous or conspiring. Things are not that simple. Each of these essays reveals the complexity of the new reproductive technologies discussion.

a massive threat to female existence rather than 'liberation' for women, as some supporters claimed it was. This was the beginning of FINNRET (Feminist International Network on the New Reproductive Technologies).

Next, a crucially important conference took place in April 1985. German feminists supported by churches, unions and a growing network of 'cripple' women advocating for their right to be alive, held a rousing Congress 'Women against Gene and Reproductive Technologies' in Bonn. More than 2000 participants issued a clear *No* to the technological take-over of women's reproduction and lives (Die Grünen im Bundestag, 1985). A risk assessment discussion was rejected – the technologies were (rightly) perceived as uncontrollable and needed to be stopped. The media was on side and so was the general public.

Months later in the same year, FINNRET convened an 'Emergency Conference' in Vållinge, Sweden. Buoyed by the events in Germany, the name of the network was changed to FINRRAGE (Feminist International Network of Resistance to Reproductive and Genetic Engineering) to better reflect the inclusion of genetics in our critique, as well as our philosophical position: we are an international women-centred network whose ultimate aim is to *stop* these dehumanising technologies rather than regulate them because we believe that they are part of women's oppression and constitute violence against women and other non-human animals and plants.

Events that year were followed by a rapid growth of FINRRAGE affiliates with chapters in more than twenty countries, intensive networking amongst the members, and more conferences in Spain, Australia, Austria, Bangladesh and Brazil as well as a second huge conference in Germany in 1988. This conference again received tremendous support from the general public in German-speaking countries who could obviously see the enormous potential for abuse of this 'weapon for social control' that vastly exceeded its supposedly beneficial uses (see Bradish, Feyerabend and Winkler, 1989).[74]

That the biggest rejection of reproductive technologies to date took place in Germany, is, of course, not surprising. Heidrun Kaupen-Haas, Director of the Institut für Medizin-Soziologie in Hamburg, has thoroughly documented the continuity of

---

74 FINRRAGE members consequently published a plethora of books internationally, e.g. Pat Spallone and Deborah Steinberg (eds.), *Made to Order*, 1987; Jocelynne Scutt (ed) *The Mother Machine* 1988/1989; Renate Klein, *The Exploitation of a Desire*, 1989a; and *Infertility: Women Speak Out about Their Experiences of Reproductive Medicine* (ed) 1989b; Farida Akhter, *Depopulating Bangladesh: Essays on the Politics of Fertility*; Robyn Rowland, *Living Laboratories: Women and Reproductive Technologies*, 1992; Janice Raymond, *Women as Wombs: Reproductive Technologies and the Battle over Women's Freedom*, 1993/1995; and Farida Akhter, *Resisting Norplant*, 1995. In 1988, we started the journal *Reproductive and Genetic Engineering: A Journal of International Feminist Analysis*, Pergamon Press (see <http://www.finrrage.org> for many of these journal articles). The importance of this literature stressing the two sides of the coin - fertility *control* of the poor via dangerous contraceptives, abortion and sterilisation, and fertility *'cures'* for the rich in westernised countries via dangerous IVF drugs - can not be overstated. In the 21st century, the shocking reality of this duality has only increased, and needs urgent discussion, especially in the context of sub-Saharan African countries which have become the latest 'playground' for population controllers who ply its women with dangerous contraceptives and chemical abortion (see Klein *et al.*, 2013, pp. lxxxvi–lxxxviii).

experimentation in Nazi Germany both to sterilise 'unworthy' women and to 'cure' infertility for those women who were required as Aryan breeders. As Kaupen-Haas puts it, "It is thus important to emphasize that the extermination of 'unworthy' forms of life and the promotion of desired forms of life are by themselves inseparable parts of this technology" (1988, p. 127).

The reproductive and genetic engineering industry as a dangerous field for the exploitation, commercialisation and industrialisation of women's reproduction, present and future, had become a feminist topic of such significance that it ranked second only to discussions of sexual violence in national and international feminist conferences. Surrogacy was a regular topic, although until the beginning of the 1990s, when the exploitation of women in poor so-called developing countries like India accelerated, with some exceptions in the UK and Australia, discussions remained mostly confined to events in the proliferating surrogate industry in the USA. In fact, the second German Congress in 1988 celebrated the successful resistance to Noel Keane's attempt to establish a surrogate agency in Frankfurt, Germany, called 'United Family International.' Keane had started supplying American women from an illustrated catalogue to sperm donors from France, Italy, Israel, Greece and Australia. In January 1988, a German Court ordered the immediate closing of Keane's business. France had already shut down three surrogate agencies in 1987. And what was, possibly, the first death of a so-called surrogate mother, happened in 1987 in the USA when Denise Mounce, 24, in a pregnancy arranged by surrogate broker Gene Search, Inc.

died in her eighth month of pregnancy (Corea and de Wit, 1988, pp. 190–191, see also below p.120).

In re-reading these first surrogacy cases in western countries, the greed of surrogate agencies to profit from media interest in 'their' pregnant breeders and so attract more customers, stands out. It continues today, unabated and constantly increasing.

In the UK in 1984, Kim Cotton, who had left school at sixteen, married young and had two children early, felt trapped by escalating debt. When she saw an American agency on TV offering £6,500 for British women to be inseminated with a man's sperm, she saw this as a way out of her problems; see *For Love and Money* (Cotton and Winn, 1985). Although she later calculated that the £6,500 amounted to less that one pound per hour, which was less than cleaners were paid, she remained happy with her decision. But Kim's relatively easy pregnancy was derailed when the agency wanted her to sign an exclusive deal with a newspaper. Tempted by the additional money, she was hunted by the media as the first paid surrogate in the UK and her life became public property.

As a consequence, after the baby was born in an agonisingly long labour which had her husband scared to death for Kim's life, the little girl had to stay alone in the hospital and became a ward of the state until, more than two weeks later, a High Court Judge decided that the 'commissioning parents' were of good standing. Baby Cotton, as the child became known, was flown out of the country by her foreign father and Kim has never heard of her fate. The agency then told her that she would not be paid, as the legal costs to 'rescue' the baby from the British state amounted to £11,000! (In the end the commissioning father had to pay the legal bill and so 'his' biological child ended up costing him £25,000.)

Already during Kim's pregnancy, the Warnock Committee (chaired by moral philosopher, Lady Mary Warnock) had decided that commercial surrogacy including surrogate agencies was to be made illegal in the UK. This law, enacted in 1985, has remained in place until today, but so-called altruistic surrogacy continues and in fact prospers.

What stands out in Kim Cotton's ghostwritten story are two points: Firstly, she says, she would never have engaged in surrogacy if she had wanted more children (her husband had undergone a vasectomy), and secondly, it was important to her that she never met the future parents of her baby and had no knowledge of who they were. Knowing their identity and/or being in touch with them, Kim felt, would have made it much harder for her to give her daughter away. This is, of course, in contrast to today's advice by surrogacy agencies and pro-surrogacy 'consumer groups' to maintain a relationship between the birth mother, her child, and her or his new family.

Meanwhile, in the USA, so-called surrogate mothers had begun to speak out against the practice of baby selling that had taken a devastating toll on their lives and families. Together with FINRRAGE members, political activist Jeremy Rifkin, Head of the Foundation of Economic Trends and his attorney Andrew Kimbrell, on 1 September 1987, they launched the National Coalition against Surrogacy. One of its founders (together with Gena Corea) was Elizabeth Kane (a pseudonym, her real first name is Mary Beth) who had been America's first legal 'surrogate' mother in 1980. Kane, who had described herself as 'just an incubator' when paraded on TV by her surrogacy doctor like an enthusiastic show pony for the cause of surrogacy, came to bitterly regret giving her son Justin away. Her book *Birth Mother* (1988/1990) details her story, reconstructed from her diaries. It becomes very clear that even during the time when she was a willing 'surrogate', those around her, IVF doctor Richard Levin, a surrogacy lawyer, and a local pastor – all of whom she trusted – exploited her confidence mercilessly for their own monetary gain and fame.

Elizabeth/Mary Beth tried to resist – she was never a 'docile' woman who agreed to everything. But she lost out every time. One particularly harrowing betrayal occurred during the birth. Kane had forbidden her doctor to allow filming the birth, but as her labour started, a photographer appeared in the birthing room. Elizabeth/Mary Beth told him to get out, but he stayed. She tried to find Richard Levin, but he had disappeared. When the contractions became too painful, the photographer was no longer her focus. So the birth was filmed. Perhaps even more shockingly, it was then later played to Kane and a live audience on the Phil Donohue Show without her having seen the footage first (p. 246).

All this happened before Margaret Atwood penned her hugely successful novel *The Handmaid's Tale* in 1985. Kane might as well have been called 'Ofrichard' in her real life drama, in the same way that the main character in Atwood's book was called 'Offred,' such was the control of her life by Richard Levin.[75]

Another heartbreaking moment occurred after the birth when Kane, still in hospital, wanted to visit her son in the nursery. Levin had promised her she could see him, but reneged – or 'forgot' to pass the request on to the nurses, as he said. Kane insisted and won. When she rang the nursery first to make sure it was a good time to visit, she was told they were ready for her, only to receive a return phone call within minutes to say, "There's been a mistake. We thought you were his mother" (p. 237). In spite of the excruciating pain, Kane insisted and was finally given the green light. But, as she got ready to enter the room, she caught a glimpse of Justin's 'father' holding her son in his arms and gazing at him, watched by his new 'mother'. She froze; turned around and walked away (p. 242):

> I made no attempt to brush away the tears that began to slide down my face. A mixture of pride and accomplishment, sorrow and love for the child I had conceived and nourished, given birth to and loved, swirled through me. I would never again have the opportunity to hold him close.

---

75 Margaret Atwood used the term 'handmaiden' rather than 'surrogate' in her 1985 book (she does mention 'surrogate mothers' in her 'Historical Notes' at the end of the book, p. 317). It is good to see that in the promotion for the 2017 TV series (which followed after an earlier film version and an opera), the term 'surrogate' is used. The US series, created by Bruce Miller, filmed in Canada and starring Elisabeth Moss, premiered in April 2017. A second series is planned for 2018.

This was indeed what happened and by the time of writing her book, she had not seen her son again. Over the years, his new 'parents' sent her some photos that showed him engaging in sports and luxury holidays, proving to Kane – a working-class woman – what a good life these rich people were giving her son.

In 1987, she called Justin's 'father' to ask if she could see her son, but was told that the child had been "... a business arrangement. I kept my end of the bargain, you've been paid, why do you feel the need to change the agreement?" (p. 265).

Kane continued to reflect (1988/1990, p. 265):

> How will I begin to explain to Justin that he was traded for the price of a new car?[76] What will I say when he asks me why I never fought for him in court? Will I ever be able to convince him that by the time I verbalized the loss of him, he was already six years old, and a lawsuit would have destroyed his emotional stability?

After a few more months with Richard Levin on the media circuit to praise surrogacy and secure him new clients, Kane couldn't continue to put fake smiles on her face. She slid into months of debilitating depression, neglecting her children and her marriage, almost resulting in a divorce. Suicidal thoughts were frequent.

---

76 Elizabeth/Mary Beth Kane received $11,500 for her son from the baby buyers. She told her husband to put it in a bank account and did not want to buy anything with the money. It only became useful when she had to pay tax to the American Government because she had a higher income in 1980 than usual (1988/1990, pp. 245–246). Similar to prostitution, this turns countries and states that have legalised surrogacy into pimps who profit from baby buying.

In the 'Epilogue' to *Birth Mother*[77] Mary Beth Kane details how she slowly overcame the depths of her despair in which she mercilessly blamed herself for being 'weak' and unable to get a grip and continue with her life.

One event that helped her on the road to recovery was an article she found published in *People Magazine* in October 1986.

She read about the plight of Mary Beth Whitehead who had given birth to baby Sara on 27 March 1986, contracted as a 'surrogate' for $10,000 by a wealthy couple, William and Betsy Stern,[78] through the Infertility Center of New York (whose founder and director was well known surrogacy lawyer, Noel Keane). After the birth, she gave Sara to the Sterns, but could not bear the loss. She was allowed to see her child, asked to have her back, and then did not return her. When five policemen came to raid her house, she handed Sara through a back window to her husband who fled with her to Florida (where Mary Beth's parents lived). Whitehead, who was in her nightgown, was handcuffed and taken away in front of her screaming children and neighbours. When she was released, she joined her daughter

---

77 In the Epilogue of the Australian edition of *Birth Mother* (1990, with a Foreword by Robyn Rowland), Mary Beth Kane details her two trips to Australia which included a public debate with Linda Kirkman in 1989 who, amidst a media frenzy, had given birth to baby Alice in 1988 in a sister-to-sister surrogacy, see pp. 122–137 below). I well remember meeting Mary Beth and being most impressed by her determined resolve to expose what surrogacy does to women and their families.

78 Betsy Stern, a paediatrician, was not infertile, but was worried that a pregnancy and birth would make her mild case of multiple sclerosis worse (in Arditti, 1988, p. 51).

for 87 days in Florida and desperately tried to find a lawyer. But because she and her family had no money (her husband worked as a garbage collector), no one was willing to represent her. Again, the police came and took baby Sara away, knocking Mary Beth's mother, who was looking after the child that day, to the ground. Her ten-year old daughter Tuesday, yet again witnessed the police violence.

After Elizabeth/Mary Beth Kane had read the story, she remembers that "A burning rage slowly spread through me as I read about her nightmare." She wrote a letter to Whitehead, "So you fell in love with your baby, Mary Beth, and no one told you it would happen? Well so did I. So do we all" (1988/1990, p. 268). *People Magazine* reprinted her letter and the Baby M case – as it would become known, because the Sterns called the baby Melissa – became international news.

On 31 March 1987, New Jersey Superior Court Judge Harvey Sorkow ruled in favour of the 'natural father' William Stern and against the 'surrogate' Mary Beth Whitehead (these are the terms Sorkow used in his judgment). Stern got custody of Baby M and Whitehead's parental rights were terminated. Sorkow also called surrogacy an 'alternative reproduction vehicle'. His character assessment of Whitehead is damning, not only is she poor and uneducated, she is also "very controlling of her children and husband ... and dominates the family. Mr Whitehead is clearly in a subordinate role ... She is manipulative, impulsive and exploitative" (in Arditti, 1988, pp. 55–56). The Sterns, on the other hand, are described as good and highly educated members of the community who will be able "... to afford music lessons and athletics ... it is expected that 'Baby M' will attend college" (in Arditti, 1988, p. 54).

Thirty years later, as so-called surrogate mothers in the USA continue to fight for the right to keep their babies (as exposed by Stop Surrogacy Now, see below, pp. 145–153 for more details), these same attributes are used: the birth mother is poorly educated, looks like she might lack mothering skills – while the baby buyers are well-to-do pillars of society (with plenty of cash to hire a fleet of lawyers).

The judgment was a win for defenders of 'procreative liberty'. As Judge Sorkow put it:

> It must be reasoned that if one has a right to procreate coitally, then one has a right to reproduce non-coitally ... this court holds that the protected means extend to the use of surrogates (in Arditti, 1988, p. 55).

Fortunately, aided by the support for Whitehead from a growing number of other birth mothers such as Kane, and feminists such as Corea, financial backing was found to appeal the case in the New Jersey Supreme Court. The Foundation for Economic Trends submitted a 45-page Amicus brief, [79] written by its lawyer Andrew Kimbrell and signed by Jeremy Rifkin and 22 feminists, many from FINRRAGE. The brief criticises Judge Sorkow's one-sided view of 'procreative liberties' for the sperm donor only, by radically depersonalising Whitehead as "a factor of conception

---

79 According to the Public Health Law Center, Amicus briefs are "legal documents filed in appellate court cases by non-litigants with a strong interest in the subject matter." For more information see <http://www.publichealthlawcenter.org/documents/resources/amicus-curiae-briefs>

and for gestation that the [Stern] couple lacks" (in Arditti, 1988, p. 57) and argues:

> Mary Beth Whitehead has a constitutionally protected right, as the biological mother, to the care, custody, and companionship of her child ... no person has a right to seek enforcement of a contract depriving another person of constitutionally protected rights (p. 57).

Whilst waiting for the outcome of the appeal, the National Coalition against Surrogacy began their work on 1 September 1987. Its aim was to set up a national support and legal network that would give free advice to birth mothers, but also canvass legislators in US states to ban surrogacy and surrogacy contracts. At the Coalition's first press conference, former 'surrogates' Alejandra Muñoz and Patricia Foster[80] spoke, as did Gena Corea who asked these pertinent questions – alas still relevant today:

> Is it in the best interest of female children to be born into a world where there is a class of breeder women? How damaging might that be to the self-esteem of girl children? If it is damaging, does that matter? ... As a society do we want to industrialize reproduction? Is absolutely everything grist for the capitalist mill? Are there any limits to what can be bought and sold? (in Arditti, 1988, p. 61).

---

80 The stories of Alejandra Muñoz, Patricia Forster, Nancy Barass, Mary Beth Whitehead and Elizabeth Kane can be found in my 1989 anthology *Infertility: Women Speak out about Their Experiences of Reproductive Medicine*, pp. 133–159. They are as raw and painful as when they were first written and should not be forgotten, especially as they are, shamefully, still repeated all over the world today.

Elizabeth/Mary Beth Kane remembers with pride how she and other birth mothers over the following years testified at congressional and state hearings and were instrumental in banning surrogacy in ten states: Louisiana, Michigan, Florida, Indiana, Kentucky, Nebraska, Utah, Arizona, Washington State and North Dakota (1988/1990, p. 279). Many more birth mothers became brave enough to go public with their stories. But it was also during this time that the first (official) death of a 'surrogate' mother happened. Denise, a woman living in Texas who was recovering from a recent divorce and was in debt, became a 'surrogate' as she badly needed money. Unfortunately, when she was six months pregnant, her doctor discovered she had a heart condition. She was told to get a heart monitor, but did not have $250 to buy one. Neither the baby broker, nor the commissioning parents, offered any assistance. In her eighth month of pregnancy she was found dead in her bed "with her unborn son nestled inside her" (in Kane, 1988/1990, p. 277).

On 3 February 1988, the New Jersey Supreme Court ruled that commercial 'surrogate' mother contracts are illegal. The Court returned parental rights to Mary Beth Whitehead. The ruling also said that surrogacy was baby selling and taking advantage of a woman's circumstances (in Arditti, 1988, p. 64).

However, it was a pyrrhic victory: the Supreme Court left custody with William Stern and so Baby M grew up in the Stern household.[81]

---

81 It is sad but not surprising to learn that on turning eighteen in 2004, Melissa Stern terminated Whitehead's parental rights and Betsy Stern adopted her.

Feminist author, Phyllis Chesler, well known for her best-selling books *Women and Madness* (1972) and *Mothers on Trial* (1987), had also joined the National Coalition against Surrogacy. In 1988, she published Mary Beth Whitehead's story: *Sacred Bond. The Legacy of Baby M* (1988). In her book, Chesler argued that surrogacy is a form of child abuse and sex discrimination and that surrogates are victims of the patriarchal system that instills the Christian tenets of female obedience, sacrifice, and subservience.

Commenting on these painful US surrogacy stories, sociologist Barbara Katz Rothman, the author of *The Tentative Pregnancy: Prenatal Diagnosis and the Future of Motherhood* (1986), in which she had asked important questions about prenatal testing influencing the relationship of the pregnant woman with her baby, put it simply: "The time to stop such nightmare visions is now" (1989, p. 237). She elaborated further:

> We stop it by not acknowledging the underlying principle of surrogate contracts, by not accepting the very concept of 'surrogacy' for motherhood. A surrogate is a substitute. In some human relations, we can accept no substitutes. Any pregnant woman is the mother of the child she bears ... we will not accept the idea that we can look at a woman, heavy with child, and say the child is not hers. The fetus is part of the woman's body, regardless of the source of the egg and sperm. Biological motherhood is not a service, not a commodity, but a relationship (1989, pp. 237–238).

As journalist Bonnie Goldstein pointedly said (Goldstein, 23 July 2009): "Big surprise, she stuck with the parents who raised her."

It is a great pity that Australian Maggie Kirkman, the egg donor to her sister Linda, who gave birth to her baby Alice on 23 May 1988, presumably did not read Barbara Katz Rothman's book – or Elizabeth Kane's – before she penned her own tome *My Sister's Child* (1989). Although Linda, the birth mother, is acknowledged as co-author, of the book's 351 pages, Linda only contributes 65 pages. (They had both been encouraged to keep diaries by their IVF doctor.)

In 1985, Maggie Kirkman, a 38-year-old highly educated upper middle-class academic and psychologist working on her PhD met her soon-to-be husband Severn from a well-known Melbourne establishment family. (We learn all about their whirlwind romance in her book.) Maggie had been married before and tried hard to have children but could not conceive. In 1978, she had to undergo a hysterectomy because of fibroids. However, her father, a medical doctor, had insisted she keep her ovaries. Severn, it turns out, is infertile, which he discovered when he wanted to become a sperm donor in 1978. This was a big blow to his self-confidence and he told no one in his family about it.

Severn suggests surrogacy only a few months' into their marriage in late 1985. Maggie describes how her jaw dropped, but how she immediately thought of her 'baby' sister Linda (1988, pp. 42–43).

Linda, eight years younger than Maggie, agrees to the idea when she hears that it would be Maggie's egg cells that were to be used rather than her own. And Maggie is quite clear that she wants the baby to be genetically hers. They talk about practical things, like the involvement of the many members of their tight-knit family. Maggie writes that no money was offered to Linda, but that of course they would pay all medical bills and also pay for a cleaner and more day care for Linda's two children. The 'tone' of events to come is set in Maggie's following remark (p. 46):

> We said we would enjoy helping Linda choose maternity clothes which we would buy for her. I have always yearned to be pregnant, not just to have children, and find pregnant women touchingly beautiful; it would be a joy to participate vicariously in Linda's pregnancy with *our* baby (my emphasis).

Maggie's 'enjoyment' and 'help' that was to engulf Linda's entire pregnancy, might be called 'control' and 'surveillance' in a different narrative.

But first a willing obstetrician had to be found: IVF surrogacy in 1985 was still rare in the world and had not been undertaken in Australia. What's more, the Victorian government had set up a committee to investigate ethical and legal aspects of IVF and related technologies. According to Maggie, it appears Professor John Leeton who had started the first IVF clinic at Monash University in Melbourne, jumped at the opportunity. When the Ethics Committee at his usual hospital turned down his request, he went to another hospital that did not have an Ethics Committee. The cheque for the embryo incubator that the hospital lacked was gladly picked up by Maggie and Severn: "... just over a thousand dollars" (p. 74). They plant a tree for The Twins (which is what they hope for) on their property and Maggie finds herself tearful: "I am obviously emotionally fragile"

(p. 76). She sleeps very little, agonises over the fate of surplus embryos (should there be any), gets stuck in bad traffic the next day (a recurring occurrence), and finds her memory "succumbing to tension and confusion" (p. 77).

It is Maggie who organises all meetings and all family members; they rush through peak-hour traffic and you can hear her stress levels going up with every page you turn. Linda meanwhile says matter-of-factly: "I like to do things to help other people. I often see a need, but don't always get around to doing anything" (p. 66).

As Maggie's uncooperative veins are pricked twice a day to measure her hormone levels – she is now on the fertility drug clomiphene citrate[82] – she waits anxiously for the IVF doctor's call later in they day. When the call is late, Maggie begins "to feel physical symptoms of panic" (p. 79) and needs all her relaxation techniques to stay calm. (The reader is beginning to need them too and we are less than a quarter of the way into the book.)

Next Maggie gets injections of hMG (human menopausal gonadotropin) that contain equal amounts of follicle-stimulating hormone (FSH) and luteinising hormone (LH). She refers to Robyn Rowland's criticism of these 'drug cocktails', but dismisses them: "I don't believe I am jeopardising my health" (p. 83).

---

82 In 1988, Robyn Rowland and I conducted an in-depth review of clomiphene citrate and its many adverse effects (Klein/Rowland, 1988), among them cardiovascular arrhythmia, chest pain, edema, hypertension, palpitations and blurred vision. In 1993, the FDA put a black box warning (the highest level) on this fertility drug when a link to ovarian cancer appeared. Sadly, it continues to be prescribed to millions of women today.

The twice-daily blood taking becomes stressful for Linda as well. The evening blood is now taken by their father (a medical doctor) as everyone has moved into their parents' house.

Drug headaches and ovary pains follow but they are all good signs, so suffering Maggie cops it on the chin and is delighted that two ultrasounds show her 'old' eggs (she is just over 40) are growing: "Illogically I felt very proud of myself ... Like a chook with a full nest I want to cluck and flap my wings" (p. 90).

After a 4 a.m. human chorionic gonadotropin (hCG) injection for Maggie, and oestrogen pills for Linda, the next step is a full anaesthetic for the egg retrieval procedure. Maggie and Severn are greatly disappointed when only two ripe eggs are extracted. As she is suffering from sore shoulders due to the gas pumped into her abdomen for the egg harvest which lasted more than an hour and a half, Maggie comments that "My feeling of being physically knocked about interacts with my anxiety over whether fertilisation will occur" (p. 96). Maggie's propensity to be a drama queen seems to be recognised within her family as Cynthia, her other sister, wryly asks: "And I suppose you have suffered more than any human being has suffered" and "And I suppose you are in agony" (p. 97).

After a long and agonising day waiting, they get the news in the evening that both eggs cells have been fertilised (the sperm donor is a family friend who remains anonymous).

The next procedure is the embryo transfer into Linda's womb with her husband Jim, as well as Maggie and Severn present in the theatre. Relief is palpable when, after more anxiety and handwringing from Maggie, a pregnancy is confirmed. The first trimester passes without too much drama except Maggie's frustration about not being in control (pp. 131–132):

> I snuffled into my hanky today because I wish I were the one who is pregnant because it's frustrating having to deal with the emotions of two women instead of one, and because I can't do much to help ease Linda's twelve weeks of 'premenstrual tension' which occur whenever she is pregnant.

Dreams about The Twins disappear when an ultrasound confirms only one embryo: "Sev and I are profoundly disappointed, in spite of knowing that we should be grateful for what we have. We continue to feel we have lost a child as I write this tonight. Was it a son or a daughter who died? Is there a son or daughter left?" (p. 137). It is Linda who points out that it will be easier for her to carry only one baby.

A solicitor reveals that it will be difficult for them to adopt Linda's baby as they are both over 40 and also, that adoption by family members is not allowed in Victoria, "except under special circumstances" on which they will have to rely (p. 129).

Maggie visits a lactation consultant as she wants to stimulate her breasts to produce breast milk. It's at that time during Linda's pregnancy, that she begins to shift from writing about 'our' baby to 'my' baby: "The thought of holding *my* baby to my breast fills me with the richest pleasure imaginable." And, "Walking away from the meeting I realised that I was talking to *my* baby as though it were in me ..." (p. 139, my emphasis).

Internalising that Linda's baby is really her baby continues when Maggie recalls a frightening thought that the baby might have Down syndrome or other genetic anomalies: "Should I take the risk of amniocentesis? It is too late to abort a baby now but should I calm my fears with knowing the truth?" (p. 148).[83]

In her diary entry (just one) during the first trimester, Linda too starts talking about "Maggie's baby" (p. 157). She feels sick a lot, is grumpy with her husband and finds it difficult teaching her reduced workload which ends at the end of the year. She defers her university studies. She has paid for her husband and daughter to travel to his parents in Scotland for five weeks around Christmas, but on his departure, her general malaise increases. But, as she writes: "Hearing from other people how wonderful I was, and that I was doing a super thing, made me feel much better" (p. 160).

It is interesting to see Linda's comment on Maggie's diary (p. 161):

> Maggie's diary is full of her emotional reactions to the pregnancy and our relationship. My diary was also supposed to record my emotional reactions to the pregnancy, but all I came up with was fatigue. I was tired and bad-tempered sometimes, but that was because I was pregnant, not because I was a surrogate mother. It occurred to me that maybe I was suppressing any emotion before it came, as a way of coping. It was not conscious, if that was the case.

Meanwhile, Maggie continues her stressed-out existence which includes being the site manager of the house they are re-building as Severn has returned to full-time work. She defers

---

83 Thirty years later, prenatal tests are seen as essential, especially with the egg donor over 40 and the pregnant woman over 30. And since 2010, abortions will be performed in Victoria virtually up to the baby's birth. Linda was lucky to escape both an amniocentesis and a potential abortion (in case of an anomaly).

her PhD for a year, as there is no time to concentrate on writing while worrying about 'her' baby and a million other activities fill her mind. Linda, meanwhile is getting grumpier by the day. As Maggie writes in her diary on 20 December 1987 (p. 173): "Today Linda said she was fed up with feeling ill, and wished that I were pregnant. She knows I share her wishes. How much simpler would it all be."

The second trimester continues with a flurry of activities of house renovating, and organising big family parties for busy Maggie, as well as continued fatigue and feeling unwell for pregnant Linda. As both Linda and Maggie live in the country-side, there are endless car journeys to 'our' medical appointments in Melbourne. New language enters the writing. The term 'gestational mother' is used for the first time by Maggie (p. 182), followed by talking about Linda and "her responsibility as an *incubator* (p. 185, my emphasis). Later, Maggie likens herself to a 'biological mother' (p. 258) and a 'gestational mother' (p. 285).

Continuing her behind-the-scenes appointments with politicians and getting more legal opinions, Maggie shows her middle-class indignation when she fumes: "Today [25 February 1988] I am agitated and angry" (p. 202). "Why should my baby have to be registered as the child of Linda and Jim?" When that appears inevitable and she learns that officially the baby will have to be put up for adoption, her answer is: "It is not what we believe we are doing and feels wrong. In our view the baby will be going to her mother, after being gestated by her aunt, she is not being given for adoption by her mother" (p. 278).

Dissociation creeps into Linda's writing. She says she does not feel ready to wear maternity clothes: "I felt as though appearing pregnant was living a lie. *I'm not having a baby, Maggie is*" (p. 214, my emphasis). And Linda's two children, talk about her mother having 'Maggie's baby' (p. 261).

As the pregnancy advances, it becomes evident that a lot of people want a piece of this 'test case'. Professor Leeton is writing a paper on what he calls "gestational surrogacy" for an IVF conference in Singapore; Monash IVF offers a media consultant (they decline). Their identity has not been revealed to the media and Maggie wants the upper hand in telling their 'real' story. A book contract (surrounded by secrecy) with Penguin Australia is signed. She intends their book to influence "the framing of laws" (p. 234) in Victoria.

The third trimester brings more driving around to medical appointments, buying Linda maternity clothes in which she looks "particularly smart" (p. 230) and higher stress levels for Maggie, not least because she is now on a three-hour per day regime to induce lactation. But also because she "collapses in a dizzy, sobbing heap"(p. 233) when it (temporarily) appears that Linda might have to look after her baby for six months until Maggie can apply for adoption: "They cannot, it seems, perceive me as the mother" (p. 231).

The bureaucratic worries that make Maggie's life a misery begin to pale into insignificance when Linda starts bleeding. She is 29 weeks' pregnant; a baby born at this age can survive, but is pre-term. Linda is taken by ambulance to a Melbourne hospital (followed by Maggie in her car). She is advised to stay in hospital for two days to see how the suspected placenta praevia (where the placenta moves closer to the cervix) is developing.[84] The ultrasound technician has revealed the sex of the baby: it's a girl. On leaving the hospital, Maggie has to walk

> past nurseries full of crying and sleeping babies. *I felt so close to my daughter that I could hardly bear to leave her among strangers.* Her strong heartbeat and obvious liveliness gave me hope, and I willed her to cling tenaciously to the safety of Linda's body (p. 240, my emphasis).

This is an extraordinary statement that shows the power of beginning to believe something that is entirely untrue. But it also shows that Maggie, with all the love she professes to have for her sister, sees her as little more than a 'body' and worries that 'her child' is left with strangers. It reinforces the arguments I made in Chapter 5 that surrogacy can not be regulated but must be stopped: feelings that can emerge during a pregnancy are completely unpredictable and can, at times, lead to great harm for one or more of the people involved.

Two days later, on 5 April 1988, an ultrasound confirms that the placenta is detaching itself from the wall of the womb and has moved into the vicinity of the cervix. (It is placenta praevia grade three, with the highest level being four.) Furthermore, the baby appears to be very small and there is a worry it might

---

84 It was not known in 1988 that a pregnancy with 'donor' eggs leads more frequently to placenta praevia (see Chapter 2, p. 29). Perhaps today Maggie would feel more 'guilty' than she did in 1988: "It would be wrong to say that I feel guilty about this turn of events. Placenta praevia occurs in one out of every 150 pregnancies and is independent of the fact that it is my baby Linda is carrying" (p. 242).

not get enough nutrients from the detaching placenta. Still in hospital, a meeting with a member of the Department of Community Services Victoria (CSV) who will assess the question of adoption takes place. Linda asserts she wants to tell him that "no one has coerced me into doing anything I don't want to do" and Maggie comments that "Linda has an advantage over me in that she is detached from the baby and seems to feel no anxiety about the baby's future" (p. 245).

Dissociation and the stress of over-investment in full display at the same time!

But more worries were to come: The baby's heart monitor showed that it was indeed not getting enough nutrients and, if not better the following day, a emergency Caesarian section would need to be performed. What's more, John Leeton rings them with the annoying news that their secret is blown and that he is busy doing interviews. So that evening they are glued to the TV hearing people talk about them – but their names have not been leaked. This appears to happen later in the day, and in the middle of the night, Linda is moved to a private hospital where no one knows the story of her baby. While Maggie recalls Linda as feeling 'teary' and 'unhappy', it is again her own distress about 'her' baby's wellbeing, and rushing around to organise everything and everybody that is centre stage.

Linda is allowed to go and stay at her parents' house in Melbourne with the hope that she will last another seven weeks and then deliver the baby by Caesarian section at 38 weeks. Maggie will stay with her the whole time: "I am now her minder for eight weeks. It's a big responsibility. I am even going to sleep with her in a double bed. Linda said it was time I was kicked in the back by the baby during the night" (pp. 253–254).

The time until the birth is filled with irritability, grumpiness, and more of Maggie's indignation about politicians who don't understand what they are doing. Maggie sticks to her sister like glue and more time is spent on trying to induce lactation in Maggie.

Linda gets to the end of her tether and cracks up sobbing. She wants to go to her home in the country. Maggie is not happy, because of worries over 'her' baby's health. A big haemorrhage on 13 May means admission by ambulance to a hospital in Melbourne. Linda wants the baby out, Maggie hopes for another week. Maggie is in a highly stressed state and, "overcome with sorrow and anxiety" (p. 264), Linda has to comfort her. The fact that placenta praevia is as dangerous for the birth mother as it is for the baby, is not mentioned.

Maggie gets her wish, but on 20 May Linda rebels: "I've had enough. I am running out of coping. There's no more patience" (p. 276). Everyone, including the reader is relieved when finally, baby Alice is born a healthy 2.4 kg via a Caesarian section on 23 May 1988. Linda, foreshadowing that she is ceasing to be of interest as everyone dashes off to be with the baby, has made sure that her husband is by her side. But this is not the end of the story yet as the two sisters spend the next few weeks together with Linda expressing breast milk for her 'niece' and Maggie feeding Alice. Two weeks' after the birth they find out that the press has discovered their names and convene an immediate press conference to present their side of the story. Linda begins:

"We wish to announce that with the help of Victoria's excellent IVF technology, I have successfully gestated my sister's baby. My niece Alice was born four weeks early on 23nd May and is thriving" (p. 336).

There are important lessons to be learned from a close re-reading of *My Sister's Child*, nearly 30 years after its publication in 1988.

The first is that no matter whether it is 'real' or a delusion, determined, educated and well-off people who are intent on acquiring a baby with (some of) their own genes, can be successful in a country or state where any form of surrogacy is permitted.

The second lesson is that two intelligent women internalised the words of wisdom from their medical expert, Professor John Leeton, whose understanding of the birth mother as a 'gestational carrier' still dominates the discourse around surrogacy today. In 1989, John Leeton explained the merits of IVF surrogacy in an interview with *New Idea* (a women's magazine):

> ... the child will be *totally theirs genetically* – her egg, his sperm – and the risk of the surrogate mother bonding to the child after that pregnancy is less ... *This is the point that everyone is missing, the vital point* (in Monks, 1989, pp. 12–13, my emphasis).

Those in the surrogacy industry who swallow Leeton's words must be mightily pleased that the hundreds of thousands of egg 'donors' around the world are not rising up to claim any child born with their genes as their own!

But the third lesson is that even wealth, connections and determination are not always sufficient to bend the rules:

Maggie Kirkman and her husband had to go to the Supreme Court to adopt her sister's child and it took fourteen months (Kirkman, 2002, p. 140). And presumably a lot of money.

Fourthly, and importantly, the Kirkman sister surrogacy was hugely supported by their close-knit large family whose members all contributed support and help during and after Linda's pregnancy. Linda herself sees Alice's conception as an "exercise of the whole extended family" (Hurley, 1989, p. 23). Elizabeth/Mary Beth Kane who came to Australia and debated Linda Kirkman at the Women's Studies Summer Institute at Deakin University on 20 January 1989, commented that

> Linda may have to suffer losses much deeper than that of her daughter Alice if she should ever reverse her position on surrogacy. Could she lose her standing within the family circle? ... I think it would be much easier for Linda to retain her current personality and continue the status quo. She would have nothing to gain from acknowledging her feelings some day (1988/1990, p. 282).[85]

And this is exactly what happened. To all intents and purposes, Alice is now a young woman close to 30 who mostly stays out of the media. But was the relationship between the sisters really as equal as Linda says it always was? Who can forget the many media appearances and stories in glossy magazines of glamourous Maggie in the latest designer outfit who glows with pride as she holds baby Alice. Nor the bow in the hair of baby

---

85 In her talk, Kane also mentioned another sister-to-sister surrogacy in the USA, where the birth mother, Lori Jean, did not want to give up her child, but was forced to by her family who then disowned her. Lori Jean had entered into the arrangement because she thought her sister would love her more for her generosity (Hurley, 1989, p. 23; Rowland, 1992, p. 69).

sister Linda (on the cover of their book and in conferences) who stands there in the photos somewhat awkwardly in a hand-knitted jumper? Like the unfussy girl who got married, moved to the countryside, worked as a school teacher and had two children who were three and five when the Baby Alice story began.

We all write our stories in the way we want our readers to understand a particular issue – my book is no exception. This means emphasising some facts rather than others. Maggie Kirkman did that by rarely referring to feminist criticism in Victoria which was at its peak in the late 1980s. When she did mention it, she dismissed it as not being pertinent to 'their' story.

The 'but-it's-different-in-our-case' mantra is another lesson to be learnt from any surrogacy cases, past or present. People who argue the merits of *their* special case put forward an individualistic rights' perspective that only has a chance of success within a country or state that situates surrogacy within a neoliberal regulatory framework. If, as I argue throughout this book, surrogacy is the taking of a baby for love or money from its birth mother after she has grown her or him from her own body, then this is a violation of a woman's bodily integrity, whatever 'consent' or 'choice' might have been invoked. There are too few good outcomes compared to the thousands of stories of heartbreak and grief, to make me reconsider my stance.

On 1 July 1988, all IVF surrogacies became illegal in the state of Victoria when the Infertility (Medical Procedures) Act 1984 was proclaimed. It stayed illegal until 1995 when the Infertility

Treatment Act became even more strict: a so-called surrogate mother had to be infertile herself before she could carry a child for other people. This put a stop to surrogacy in Victoria. The IVF industry, predominantly situated in Melbourne at that time, bemoaned the end of a new lucrative market, but had to abide by the state law. Professor Leeton is quoted as being exasperated by the 1995 law change: "This ridiculous situation effectively outlaws IVF surrogacy which was probably its overall intention" (in Milburn, 23 May, 1998).

So-called altruistic surrogacy became legal again in Victoria on 1 January 2010 when the Assisted Reproductive Technology Act 2008 came into force. It repealed the Infertility Treatment Act 1995. The 2008 Act allows for a Substitute Parentage Order to be applied for by the commissioning parents to the County or Supreme Court, a minimum of 28 days after the child is born. Once the Substitute Parentage Order has been made by the court, a new birth certificate will be issued and the 'new' parents can select a new name for the baby. It is up to the commissioning parents to tell the child of their birth mother's existence or not.

This is how, in the 21st century, a real live woman who grew a child for nine months in her womb and gave birth to it, is legally disappeared.[86]

Of course this current legal situation would have made life much easier for Maggie Kirkman in 1988 but it was not to be.

---

86 Even if the birth mother's details are saved by the registry office and can be accessed by the child when s/he reaches eighteen, it creates a similar situation to that of adoptees. Some children created by surrogacy arrangements will be desperate to find their birth mother with all the ups and downs this entails. And what about the egg 'donor' if there was one?

In a 2002 paper that Kirkman wrote about Linda's pregnancy and birth, I was astounded to read a comment by her father Jack. In her book and elsewhere (1988, p. 42; 2002, p. 137), Maggie states that she herself had come to terms with infertility after her hysterectomy, and that it had been her new husband Severn (who was infertile as well), who had come up with the idea of IVF surrogacy. Following on from this, at Alice's first birthday party, Maggie quotes her father as emphasising "... the essential contribution of Sev's lateral thinking and remembers him as saying: *'Alice is the child of Sev's brain and imagination'* " (2002, p. 142, my emphasis).

So there we have it, as I have said previously (p. 27 and p. 28), at the end of the day, it is really *men* who make babies.

Delusion rules: First we had the birth mother who said her child was not her child but her niece. Then we had the sister who was convinced that the baby was not only her child, but was actually in her body (p. 139). And now we have it confirmed that the 'brain and imagination' of the social father, who was not even the sperm donor, created the child. This is postmodernism gone wild, or The Rule of the Father aka Patriarchy having a good laugh. No wonder that The Hague Conference on Private International Law (HCCH) is focusing on parentage issues (see Chapter 5, pp. 88–91).

After the Kirkman 'experiment' in the late 1980s, surrogacy ceased to be of great media interest.[87] On 22–23 February 1991,

---

87 In the same year there was another IVF surrogacy in Australia. It was in Perth, Western Australia, where triplets, two girls and a boy, were born on 18 October 1988. The IVF doctor was Dr John Yovich. Compared to the

a National Conference was held in Melbourne: 'Surrogacy in Whose Interest?' Speakers, ranging from politicians and bureaucrats and Linda Kirkman to relinquishing mothers, bioethicists and high profile feminists, concluded by saying *No* to all surrogacy (Meggitt, ed 1991; of course Linda Kirkman disagreed). In her conference summary, Wendy Weeks, the Head of Social Work at Melbourne University put it this way:

> In sharing our experiences and knowledge there has emerged a strong view that surrogacy situations (whether commercial or supposedly altruistic) are undesirable, risky, potentially damaging social experiments and *'fabrications'* which should not be institutionalised (Meggitt (ed) 1991, p. 137, my emphasis).

Nevertheless, in 1997, the Family Court of Australia had to deal with its first custody case after surrogacy. This was a 'traditional' surrogacy in a private agreement in Queensland where two close female friends (both married, one of the couples infertile) had agreed to 'altruistic' surrogacy. But in the end, after Mrs S had handed baby Evelyn to Mrs Q, the wife of the commissioning couple, she came to bitterly regret her decision. The Family Court decided that despite having lived with Mrs Q and her husband for a year, baby Evelyn would be better off with her birth mother, Mrs S, and should be handed back.

In other developments, in 1988, the federal government convened the National Bioethics Consultative Committee

---

Victorian Kirkman surrogacy, this birth attracted far less publicity (*Canberra Times*, 20 October 1988). In 1986, a Western Australian government committee had recommended that surrogacy be prohibited, but no legislation had been passed.

(NBCC), who in 1992 recommended to Parliament that 'altruistic' surrogacy should be legalised but with strict conditions, e.g. the birth mother should be given a 'cooling off' period of one month. However, the Committee's recommendations were ignored and the NBCC was disbanded. Two of its members, science lecturer, Heather Dietrich, and scientist, Sister Regis Dunne, had written Dissenting Reports to the Committee's Majority Report, in which Dunne said, rather bluntly:

> I am not convinced that the legal establishment of surrogacy will prevent informal private arrangements, nor do I think state licensed agencies could successfully screen applicants nor ensure harms will not be done. *The best way to prevent harm is not to engage in the practice at all* (in Meggitt, ed 1991, p. 133, my emphasis).

I could not agree more and this remains my view in 2017.

Meanwhile, in 1989, Canada had established a Royal Commission on Reproductive Technologies with Patricia Baird as its Chair. After spending 28 million dollars of taxpayers' money (in Munro, 1997, p. 332), the Commission issued its final report 'Proceed with Care' in 1993. In spite of the input of many feminists and FINRRAGE members, the report recommended regulation, not abolition. Still, commercial surrogacy and the buying and selling of sperm, eggs and embryos was to be prohibited, as was ectogenesis and sex selection. But when the Bill drafted from the Commission's findings was tabled in Parliament in 1993, it was not voted on as the Parliament was dissolved. Since then there have been a number of attempts to regulate the IVF industry, but no overarching regulation has ever been achieved (Norris and Tiedeman, 2011). Nevertheless, in

2017, commercial surrogacy remains prohibited, but 'altruistic' surrogacy is allowed. In fact, Canada has become an attractive destination country for Australians seeking cross-border surrogacy.

Around the world, more feminist conferences were held and books produced; for example *Sortir la maternité du laboratoire* in Québec, Canada, in 1988, and *L'ovaire-dose?* in Paris in 1989 (Lesterpt and Doat, 1989).

The culmination of FINRRAGE members' activities to date came to fruition at a 1989 conference in Bangladesh whose Proceedings became known as *The Declaration of Comilla* (Akhter *et al.*, 1989). For more than a week, 149 participants from 34 countries met in a rural area. The conference was hosted by FINRRAGE member and Director of UBINIG, Farida Akhter.[88] Bangladesh was chosen because we wanted women from western countries meeting with their sisters from poorer nations on their land in order to understand similar and different problems that confronted us. In the spirit of FINRRAGE, it was

---

88 UBINIG (Policy Research for Development Alternative) is a community based and community led research and advocacy organisation in Bangladesh, linking life, ecology and livelihood strategies of communities for dignity, diversity and the joy of living; <http://ubinig.org/index.php/home/index/english> It has become internationally renowned for its concept of 'Nayakrishi Andolon'. This translates to 'new agricultural movement' which resists the economic and technological processes that is turning the earth into barren fields and industrial deserts. UBINIG supports thousands of farmers in villages throughout Bangladesh in which pesticide-free organic food is produced, women are important keepers of seeds, and the communities also resist social ills such as dowries and harmful contraceptives forced on poor women.

crucial for us to link pro-natalist technologies such as IVF and surrogacy with anti-natalist policies such as population control via harmful contraceptives, sex selection and sterilisation. Surrogacy was discussed and rejected (see also Klein, 2008, pp. 160–162). Paragraph 28 of *The Declaration of Comilla* reads as follow (Akhter *et al.*, 1989, p. x): [89]

> We condemn any national and international traffic in women, eggs and embryos, human organs, body parts, cells or DNA especially for purposes of reproductive prostitution which exploits women as human incubators, in particular poor women and women in poor countries. We also strongly protest against the existence of 'baby farms' and commercial adoption and surrogacy agencies.

The Comilla conference was an important contribution to building solidarity between women from many different parts of the world and sent us all home greatly enriched and more determined to do whatever we could to stop these dehumanising technologies. Theresia Degener, a German woman whose mother took Thalidomide, astonished people in Comilla, as she carried her bags on her shoulders and ate with a fork between her toes (she has no arms). Degener, who has since become a law professor in Germany, exemplified one of FINRRAGE'S most important maxims: all life is worthwhile and prenatal testing will do more harm than good. As she put it: "... disability is another way of life and society needs to create enough scope

---

89 *The Declaration of Comilla* (Akhter *et al.*, 1989) can be accessed here; <http://ubinig.org/index.php/campaigndetails/showAerticle/15/23/english>):

and facilities for such a life to be lived well" (in Akhter *et al.*, 1989, p. 165).

A further bonus was that over 80 participants from Asian countries (Philippines, Japan, India and Indonesia) established an 'Asian FINRRAGE hub' and met again in 1990 for a FINRRAGE-UBINIG Regional Meeting.

The next international FINRRAGE Congress 'Women, Procreation, and Environment', was held in Rio de Janeiro, Brazil, from 30 September to 7 October 1991. It was in part a preparatory meeting for the 1994 NGO Forum at the International Conference on Population and Development (ICPD) which showcased an 'International Public Hearing on Crimes against Women Related to Population Policies' (Klein, 2008, p. 164). A year before, UBINIG had yet again hosted an important international meeting against population control policies: People's Perspectives on 'Population' Symposium.

After these events, new international challenges arose such as the cloning of Dolly the sheep in 1996 that opened up a novel frontier for critics opposed to genetic engineering and tinkering with the production of life, be it animal or human. The next decade saw governments around the world debate legislation on embryonic stem cell research which could not be undertaken without bought or 'donated' eggs from women. As I have already mentioned earlier (Chapter 2, pp. 18–19), in 2006, concerned feminists joined in the international network Hands Off Our Ovaries (HOOO), pointing – yet again – to the serious dangers to women from the process of 'donating' eggs. In 2010, the US Center for Bioethics and Culture produced its extraordinary documentary 'Eggsploitation' (see Chapter 2, p. 15 and pp. 20–21) that exposed short- and long-term health problems, including cancer suffered by women who had agreed to provide eggs for infertile couples or research. The documentary also includes medical specialists who are critical of this practice.

The first decade of the 21st century saw the quick rise of India and other poor countries in the so-called Third World as cheap surrogacy destinations for international baby buyers which included a new group of wealthy clients: gay men. Many countries started to get worried about these exploding markets which were, clearly, leading to the exploitation of women and children. On 5 April 2011, the European Parliament adopted a 'resolution on priorities and outline of a new EU policy framework to fight violence against women' in which these two paragraphs on surrogacy were included:

20. Asks Member States to acknowledge the serious problem of surrogacy which constitutes an exploitation of the female body and her reproductive organs;

21. Emphasizes that women and children are subject to the same forms of exploitation and both can be regarded as commodities on the international reproductive market, and that these new reproductive arrangements, such as surrogacy, augment the trafficking of women and children and illegal adoption across national boarders;

On 16 December 2015, The European Parliament accepted a motion on the Annual Report on Human Rights and Democracy in the World 2014 and the European Union's policy on the matter including the following paragraph referring to surrogacy:

114.   Condemns the practice of surrogacy, which undermines the human dignity of the woman since her body and its reproductive functions are used as a commodity; considers that the practice of gestational surrogacy which involves reproductive exploitation and use of the human body for financial or other gain, in particular in the case of vulnerable women in developing countries, shall be prohibited and treated as a matter of urgency in human rights instruments;

It is great to see the European Parliament showing leadership in attempting to stop the dehumanising practice of cross-border surrogacy. And as mentioned in Chapter 5 (p. 99), on 23 March 2015, a group of mostly European Women's Organisations headed by CoRP (Le Collectif pour le Respect de la Personne) sent a powerful document to the Hague Conference on Private International Law (HCCH) in which they demanded an International Convention for the Abolition of Surrogacy (see Chapter 5, pp. 99–102).

On 1 February 2016, some of the same groups organised a conference in Paris 'For the Universal Abolition of Surrogate Motherhood' ('Vers l'abolition de la GPA', Gestation pour Autrui). Conference participants included French politicians and European feminist authors such as Kajsa Ekis Ekman, Julie Bindel, Eva-Maria Bachinger[90] and Sheela Saravanan. The organisers described the aim of the conference as working towards the universal abolition of surrogate motherhood by bringing together

---

90   Eva Maria Bachinger's book *Kind auf Bestellung* (*Child to Order*) had been published in Austria in 2015.

politicians from all over Europe as well as feminist and human rights organizations, and researchers from various fields, in order to throw light on and fight against the unjust practice of surrogacy, which infringes on fundamental human rights.

The Conference concluded with signing The International Convention for the Abolition of Surrogacy.

As this laudable opposition to surrogacy was becoming stronger in European countries, it became clear that for critics located in different parts of the world, a new international organisation that focused on stopping both egg 'donation' and surrogacy was sorely needed. Inspired by Jennifer Lahl's sterling leadership and hard work, in May 2015, a group of 500 women and men from around the world came together to create the campaign Stop Surrogacy Now (SSN).[91]

Since its beginning in May 2015, SSN has blossomed to over international 8000 supporters (Lahl, pers. com., July 2017). Original signatories include many of the 'old' FINRRAGE feminists and other activists from the 1980s, but also 'surrogate' mothers, children born from surrogacy and/or 'donor' gametes, human rights activists, lawyers, Members of Parliament, policy makers, LGBTI activists, academics, authors, journalists, children's rights activists, adoption critics as well as prostitution survivors and organisers against violence against women. Twenty-one organisations, many of them from Europe, also

---

91 The US Center for Bioethics and Culture (CBC, which hosts SSN) had produced its second documentary 'Breeders: A Subclass of Women?' in 2014. This documentary has become an important campaign tool. Its director, Jennifer Lahl, was a paediatric critical care nurse for 25 years.

signed on, among them the Swedish Women Doctors' Society, the European Women's Lobby (Belgium), EMMA (Germany), The Women's Bioethics Alliance (Australia), FINRRAGE (Australia), Scandinavian Human Rights Lawyers, Se Non Ora Quando – Libere (Italy), Make Mothers Matter (France).

Aiming to invite a wide audience to join our efforts to raise critical awareness about the global surrogacy industry so it can be abolished, this is the text of the SSN statement (available in German, English, Spanish, French, Italian, Japanese, Norwegian and Swedish):

Stop Surrogacy Now Statement

We are women and men of diverse ethnic, religious, cultural, and socio-economic backgrounds from all regions of the world. We come together to voice our shared concern for women and children who are exploited through surrogacy contract pregnancy arrangements.

Together we affirm the deep longing that many have to be parents. Yet, as with most desires, there must be limits. Human rights provide an important marker for identifying what those limits should be. We believe that surrogacy should be stopped because it is an abuse of women's and children's human rights.

Surrogacy often depends on the exploitation of poorer women. In many cases, it is the poor who have to sell and the rich who can afford to buy. These unequal transactions result in consent that is under informed if not uninformed, low payment, coercion, poor health care, and severe risks to the short- and long-term health of women who carry surrogate pregnancies.

The medical process for surrogacy entails risks for the surrogate mother, the young women who sell their eggs, and the children born via the assisted reproductive technologies employed. The risks to women include Ovarian Hyper Stimulation Syndrome (OHSS), ovarian torsion, ovarian cysts, chronic pelvic pain, premature menopause, loss of fertility, reproductive cancers, blood clots, kidney disease, stroke, and, in some cases, death. Women who become pregnant with eggs from another woman are at higher risk for pre-eclampsia and high blood pressure.

Children born of assisted reproductive technologies, which are usually employed in surrogacy, also face known health risks that include: preterm birth, stillbirth, low birth weight, fetal anomalies, and higher blood pressure. A surrogate pregnancy intentionally severs the natural maternal bonding that takes places in pregnancy—a bond that medical professionals consistently encourage and promote. The biological link between mother and child is undeniably intimate, and when severed has lasting repercussions felt by both. In places where surrogacy is legalized, this potential harm is institutionalized.

We believe that the practice of commercial surrogacy is indistinguishable from the buying and selling of children. Even when non-commercial (that is, unpaid or 'altruistic'), any practice that subjects women and children to such risks must be banned.

No one has a right to a child, whether they are heterosexual, homosexual, or single-by-choice.

We stand together asking national governments of the world and leaders of the international community to work together to end this practice and **Stop Surrogacy Now**.

<http://www.stopsurrogacynow.com>

During the past two years, representatives from SSN have testified at US states' hearings into surrogacy, supported 'surrogate' mothers' legal fights to keep their children, and organised, or participated in, important meetings, e.g. conferences in New York, Rome and Madrid.[92]

SSN is also increasingly approached by birth mothers (not just from the US but also from Canada, the UK and Australia) who have been greatly harmed during surrogacy (commercial or 'altruistic'), carry unreasonable financial burdens, or who want their children back. This is not easy as these women need lawyers and counsellors and the US Center for Bioethics and Culture is a not-for-profit organisation. But it is obvious that similar to the needs of prostitution survivors, the ills that women and their children suffer in this exploitative global industry, are huge. Their needs are substantial and their numbers are increasing.

SSN, and in particular, Jennifer Lahl, has also exposed the 'myth' promulgated by the pro-surrogacy lobby in Australia and visiting US IVF doctors (especially those from California), that in the USA, surrogacy is well regulated and no problems exist. Just as in other countries, the health of 'surrogates' and egg 'donors' can be greatly affected, sometimes for life. (This is documented in 'Maggie's story', who talks about her fight against

---

92   The list of SSN activities to-date can be found on the Stop Surrogacy Now webpage <http://www. stopsurrogacynow.com> under Resources which also includes a good list of books and articles critical of surrogacy as well as some films. (A book with personal stories by women who were engaged as 'altruistic' or commercial 'surrogate' mothers is in preparation; Lahl and Tankard Reist, 2018.)

advanced breast cancer after egg 'donation', and the other two films mentioned earlier, 'Eggsploitation' and 'Breeders'.) Other recent upsetting stories include 'surrogate' mother Brooke Browne's death in Idaho from late pregnancy complications when carrying twins for a couple in Spain (the babies died too); the protracted custody battle of Californian 'surrogate' Melissa Cook who refused to abort one of the three foetuses she was carrying; and Brittneyrose Torres who was also carrying triplets and required many weeks of hospitalisation due to pregnancy complications (in Lahl, 2016).

Of course, these upsetting stories represent only a small part of what we know. We must not forget that the baby buyers will always have more money at their disposal than the 'surrogates' when it comes to legal or unpaid medical costs. Because the IVF industry in the USA is completely unregulated, there are no state or national bodies that collect statistics on these unfortunate events. There is no medical, legal and other support available from the surrogacy agencies or baby brokers who always side with the paying customers. It is thus a *gross* misrepresentation to call surrogacy in the USA 'well regulated' and without problems.

Returning to Stop Surrogacy Now, I will only briefly mention three recent campaign events:[93]

1. On 14 March 2017, SSN held a workshop as part of the UN Commission on the Status of Women 'Trading on the Female

---

93 For more details about the SSN campaign see <http://www.stopsurrogacy now.com/conference-in-rome-surrogacy-a-real-dehumanization-of-mother-and-child/#sthash.J4doYYcV.Lq8B4Hh3.dpbs> The FINRRAGE and SSN Facebook pages are other sites for campaign details.

Body'. The two hour session included presentations by Jessica Kern, a young woman born from a surrogacy arrangement, who refers to herself as a 'product; 'surrogate' mother Kelly, who undertook three commercial surrogacies including giving birth to twins for a French gay couple when she was 20, and twins for a Spanish heterosexual couple (surrogacy is illegal in both countries), and Kylie, who sold her eggs and had serious health problems including a stroke from ovarian hyperstimulation syndrome (OHSS). This led to permanent eye and memory problems and likely impaired fertility. The panel also included anti-surrogacy critics, *Guardian* journalist Julie Bindel, ethicist Professor Janice Raymond and Pierrette Pape, Policy and Campaigns Director of the European Women's Lobby.

Kelly's story, in particular, is one of a repeated series of gross deception and exploitation and will be featured in a forthcoming new documentary by Jennifer Lahl.[94]

2. On 23 March 2017, at its international meeting in Rome, the feminist group Se Non Ora Quando? – Libere (If Not Now When – Free), original signatories to SSN, presented a request to the United Nations, Human Rights Treaties Division, to address surrogacy in the Convention on the Elimination of All Forms of Discrimination against Women (CEDAW):

> We, signers, request the United Nations bodies, in charge of honouring the Convention on the Elimination of All Forms

---

94 The two-hour video of the UN event can be watched here: <http://www.stopsurrogacynow.com/what-a-great-event/#sthash.ddOcirOD.cSO3gXSQ.dpbs>

of Discrimination against Women (CEDAW) on child and human rights, to create a procedure aimed at recommending the practice of surrogate motherhood to be prohibited, as incompatible with the respect of human rights and women's dignity.

And further:

8.   Therefore, it becomes necessary to involve UN agencies to start building up the conditions to abolish surrogate motherhood at the international level. In this regard, it is urgent to adopt – in the framework of the CEDAW – a recommendation against surrogate motherhood on the model of the one adopted to fight female genital mutilation practices. This option reaches the widest consensus in the process leading to its universal abolition.

In the resolution, read at the meeting, the signers point out that they

don't have to fall into the rhetorical trap of individual freedom and 'the wonderful gift of life'. Surrogate motherhood leads to a real dehumanization of mother and child as it consciously creates a state of sacrifice and abandonment. The desire of becoming a parent can't be raised to an individual right for the 'customer' in order to take control over a woman's body and consequently making a child's life a private property.

It will be interesting to see how the United Nations deals with this request.

3. On 26 April 2017, a group of SSN Campaigners called for the abolition of surrogacy in Spain and showed the documentary 'Breeders' (translated into Spanish as 'Criadoras: Una Clase

inferior de mujeres?'). The group, consisting of Jennifer Lahl, former 'surrogate' Kelly Martinez, Pierrette Pape from the European Women's Lobby, UK journalist, Julie Bindel, and UK LGBTI activist, Gary Powell, addressed Spanish Members of Parliament and met with the newly formed Spanish anti-surrogacy group Red Estatal Contra El Alquiler de Vientres, highlighting the harms of surrogacy. Kelly's story, as already mentioned above (pp. 149–150) was particularly harrowing.

Unbeknownst to Kelly, the Spanish commissioning couple had paid extra money for her to be implanted with an XX (female) embryo and a XY (male) embryo. However, the female embryo did not develop, and the male embryo spontaneously divided so that she ended up carrying twin boys. The baby buyers were furious when they were informed of this development after an ultrasound. They treated Kelly so badly that her stress and blood pressure levels rose dangerously and she ended up seriously ill with pre-eclampsia. The Spanish couple picked up the babies after the Caesarian section and Kelly has not heard from them since. Nor did they pay her substantial medical bills as their US contract had included no such provision. As the SSN website puts it succinctly: "Kelly's story, not an exception in the US, shows the reality of surrogacy: a business where the consumer mentality leads to consider women as vessels and children as products."[95]

---

95 'International Campaign in Spain to call for Abolition of Surrogacy'; <http://www.stopsurrogacynow.com/international-campaigners-in-spain-to-call-for-abolition-of-surrogacy/#sthash.pOPie3D8.DcZ3OtuD.dpbs>

Gary Powell from the UK, an original signatory to SSN who is a gay man opposed to surrogacy, met with a Spanish gay man who had written a powerful article condemning the increasing numbers of gay men believing they have a right to their own child as 'Los Vientres de Alquilar: La cara mas brutal del "Gaypitalismo"' ('Wombs for Rent: The most brutal face of "Gaypitalism"'). In the article, Raul Solis condemns gay men for exploiting women, thus betraying years of solidarity when homosexuality was still a crime and lesbian and heterosexual feminists were supporting gay men (Solis, 25 March, 2017). The article features a powerful graphic: a barcode on a woman's pregnant belly.

Both Solis and Powell need to be congratulated for their stance. Indeed it is vital that gay men in other countries come out publicly to oppose the practice of surrogacy. Too often, heterosexual critics are hesitant to speak out against the powerful lobby of gay men demanding surrogacy for fear of being seen as homophobic. Women are not exploited and commodified as 'surrogates' by 'gay' or 'heterosexual' males: they are exploited by *men*.

As I hope to have shown in this chapter, both past and present resistance to global surrogacy was – and remains – powerful. But pro-surrogacy forces are formidable. Not only do they have the weight and monetary power of an unscrupulous customer-seeking multi-billion fertility industry behind them, they operate within a neoliberal market economy in which barcoded bellies of women (and the 'products' that will be removed from them) are, after the sex exploitation industries of pornography, prostitution and stripping, the latest frontier of violence against women. These 'pimps' are aided and abetted by baby buyers (gay and straight) who have turned their *desire* for a child, firstly into a *need*, and secondly into a *right*. Neoliberals and libertarians (feminists included), as always wrongly believe that salvation lies in regulation.

I fervently hope that Stop Surrogacy Now and other activist networks around the world will go from strength to strength to rebut this dehumanising violence against women and children.

In the Conclusion I will look at some 'Background' ramifications of reprogenetics for women, and offer some more thoughts on resistance.

Conclusion
Stop surrogacy now

What I have covered so far in this book is just the tip of the iceberg. For every birth mother or egg 'donor' who suffered physically and/or emotionally, for every female partner of a heterosexual couple who felt like a complete failure holding a newborn baby that is not her own, for every child from surrogacy that was given away and might be looking for their birth mother in years to come, there are thousands more around the world whose stories we will never hear. In every ongoing court case, whether it is by a birth mother to get custody of her child, or be reimbursed for pregnancy costs that the baby buyers did not pay, untold stress and misery will unfold (and lawyers will get rich). The onus will always be on the birth mother or egg 'donor' to 'prove' their claims, as surrogacy contracts (even if not enforceable as in 'altruistic' surrogacies) – as well as existing laws around the world – are stacked in favour of the 'intended parents', the baby buyers.

We also must never forget that the story of surrogacy is that of a neoliberal capitalist multi-billion industry which appears to be growing by the day, and to which 'morals' and 'ethics' matter very little, as long as (big) money can be made. With every country or (state) that closes its borders, a new destination country (or state) comes on line. Go on the internet and you will be flooded with slick promotional video clips that make the 'surrogacy' journey sound so simple, so joyful, and so full of goodwill with wonderful selfless 'surrogates' and egg 'donors'. This is of course a lesson learnt from IVF clinics who have long sold holiday packages to entice prospective clients. "Move over Thailand, Cairns is about to become a centre for medical tourism so if you're contemplating undergoing IVF why not tie it in with a holiday to the tropical north?" was a 2016 advertisement by an accommodation chain for Australia's Far North Queensland and the Great Barrier Reef (<https://www.fnqapartments.com/blog/details/Medical-Tourism-comes-to-Cairns-68>).

If Australia doesn't suit, Kiran Fertility Services offers packages to both Kenya and Ukraine (<http://surrogacydoctor.blogspot.com.au/2017/04/kiran-fertility-services-launches.html>); you can even send your frozen embryos to Kenya, should you have any. Kiran Fertility Services also guarantees egg 'donors' of your choice: African, Caucasian or Asian.

In case we need confirmation that surrogacy is baby selling and reproductive prostitution, we have to go no further than the website for La Vita Nova, a surrogacy clinic in Kiev, Ukraine. Here a young couple with a wad of Euros in the man's hands sit opposite a standing woman showing them her exposed naked belly (<http://lavitanova.net/index.php/en/independent-search-for-a-surrogate-mother>). Another of the many surrogacy clinics in Ukraine is BioTexCom which on its website says it "tops the list of leading centers for the treatment of infertility with the help of assisted methods of reproductive medicine." (Google 'Surrogacy in Ukraine' and you get 213,000 results in 0.32 seconds.)

BioTexCom shows advertisements and pictures on its website from its presence at the Australian outfit 'Families Through Surrogacy' Conferences on 11 March 2017 in London, and 12 March 2017 in Dublin, adding that the company gained many new clients from these conferences and now boasts 5000 Twitter followers (<http://biotexcom.com/biotexcom-families-surrogacy-conference-2017/>).

How is it possible, those of us living in Australia have to ask, that Families Through Surrogacy (with Sam Everingham at the helm) not only runs these lucrative yearly overseas conferences, but then, for their Australian conferences, re-imports guest speakers and their advertising packages from surrogacy clinics around the world? To repeat what I said earlier, commercial surrogacy remains prohibited throughout Australia (except the Northern Territory that has no laws, see pp. 72–73). In Queensland, New South Wales and the Australian Capital Territory *going overseas for surrogacy constitutes a criminal act and is punishable with jail.*

I suggest that this is what *soliciting* for reproductive tourism looks like and middlemen such as Families Through Surrogacy should be *banned* under any new legislation. It is they who immorally keep kindling the hopes of people who, often after ten or more IVF treatments appear defeated, yet still yearn for 'our own baby' whether 'made in Australia' or overseas. Families Through Surrogacy offer their clients happy 'surrogates' and egg 'donors' without considering that surrogacy, at its core, constitutes exploitation of two other human beings which can, and does, go horribly wrong. And no doubt, they get paid handsomely for these 'referrals' by their favourite clinics from around the world.

Cambodia is the latest case in point. On 20 November 2016, former Australian nurse and owner of Fertility Solutions, a surrogacy clinic in Phnom Penh, Tammy Davis-Charles was arrested for human trafficking and allegedly falsifying documents such as birth certificates. (She is still in jail and her court case will be decided in early August 2017.) It is noteworthy that in Australian media coverage immediately following Ms Davis-Charles' arrest (as well as follow-up stories), Mr Everingham from Families Through Surrogacy provided commentary. He appeared to be extremely well informed about details of Fertility Solutions: how many Australian couples' babies are now in limbo (between 30 and 40), how much the 'intended parents' paid (between $30,000 and $40,000) as well as pointing out that "Ms Davis-Charles was well trusted by many who had succeeded in having surrogate babies (sic) throughout her care" (in Barker, 21 November 2016,). Everingham also gave us a new term by pointing out that many couples "already have *embryos in utero*" (Barker, my emphasis). I presume he is referring to the live real and poor Khmer women whose bodies surround their wombs and whose lives, after Davis-Charles' arrest, were thrown into chaos as their payments were stopped. Question: how is it that Families Through Surrogacy has such intimate knowledge of Davis-Charles' business dealings? Everingham is quoted as saying that "while he does not condone such behaviour ["operating against the law"], many couples currently waiting on surrogate babies could lose tens of thousand dollars and the chance of a child, if her clinic was forced to stop" (Barker, 21 November 2016; see also Barker, 23 February 2017). I suggest there should be an official inquiry into all 'advice' that Family Through Surrogacy provides to their clients and whether these are really only the actions of "a consumer-based non-profit organisation focused on bringing together surrogates, intended parents and families through surrogacy to network, share their stories and stay informed about best practice in surrogacy arrangements" (from Families Through Surrogacy website, accessed 22 July 2017).

In 2017, not only did Families Through Surrogacy run their annual two-day 'global' conference in Melbourne on 3–4 June, they will also hold one-day meetings in Melbourne, Perth, Sydney and Brisbane in October. Business must be splendid and customers aplenty. (And in between you can meet them on 12 August in Stockholm, Sweden; a country whose Parliament is considering prohibiting *all* surrogacy, see Chapter 5, pp. 86–87). Of course there is always a new destination to be touted: apart from Ukraine and Canada, this October it will be Oregon with 'Surro Connexions: Compassion, Hope and the Miracle of Life', but also Greece with the 'Mediterranean Fertility Institute' in Chania, Crete – another place to combine surrogacy with a wonderful holiday. Surrogacy in Greece can only be altruistic and is not allowed for gay or single men; <https://www.ivfgreece.com/about-us/our-team/133-shirley>

Mentioning Greece brings up another, potentially huge and frightening problem. For years, Greece, a poor member state of the European Union, has been struggling with high unemployment, but also a big influx of refugees from the political trouble spots in Iraq, Kurdistan, Syria and Turkey. We know that in many countries like Germany, poor refugee women are 'absorbed' into brothels. Will we soon hear stories of them being recruited as egg 'donors' and 'surrogates' in spite of most European countries prohibiting all forms of surrogacies?

At some point we need to stop and think. We keep being smothered by this 'Foreground' news. Every day there is another sad story to report, another birth mother hurt, or dead, another egg 'donor' diagnosed with cancer. It is hard to keep up. Only occasionally is there good news. While it is very important to keep a watch on new developments in egg 'donation' and surrogacy – which is what Stop Surrogacy Now campaigners do so well – we must also scrutinise the 'Background': what is it that underlies these dizzying tales of exploiting women?[96]

When early IVF technology was expanding throughout the 1980s, feminists were often asking *why* these technologies were developing. The 'Foreground' version was, and is, of course that they were designed to alleviate the pain of infertility and make babies for desperate couples. So one easy answer to the question

---

96 US philosopher Mary Daly uses the concepts of 'Foreground' and 'Background' (drawing on Denise Connors) in her inspiring book *Gyn/Ecology: The Metaethics of Radical Feminism* (1978). Janice Raymond developed it further in *A Passion for Friends: Toward a Philosophy of Female Affection* (1986) where she talks about 'short-sight' and 'long-sight' seeing. It is a very useful tool when discussing complex issues.

'why' was "to start an international fertility industry and make billions" (which has come true). But there were, and are, more sinister grounds.

As I have already pointed out in Chapters 2 and 6, new reproductive technologies are used to literally 'cut up' real live women into our eggs and wombs, treat us with invasive danger-ous hormonal drug cocktails, and, in surrogacy, psychologically manipulate us to believe the myth that gestating a baby without a genetic connection will not cause us to feel any attachment, and hence these 'surrogate' babies are not our 'real' children.

This man-made *compartmentalising* ideology creates *Test-Tube Women*. The idea is that 'playing God' (as 1980s critics of reprotechs were wont to say) continues the 6,000 years of patriarchal domination of women[97] in which two points were, and are, central: One, men cannot gestate life and give birth to children (necessary to continue the species Homo sapiens). Two, men as a social group *loathe* women and our bodies for this power.[98] Conversely, when women 'fail' to reproduce, the disdain expressed is stark: Think about medical terms such as 'premature ovarian failure', 'hostile mucus', 'incompetent cervix',

---

97 There is widespread evidence for setting the beginnings of patriarchy at around 6,000 years ago. For excellent Timelines on pre-patriarchal history see Judy Foster's *Invisible Women of Prehistory: Three million years of peace, six thousand years of war* (2013). See pp. ix-xiii and the Timelines that begin Chapters 11-16 in Part III.

98 Of course this only applies to women who 'should' procreate. Poor, non-western, non-mainstream 'ethnic' women and women with disabilities who should not reproduce, are attacked with dangerous long-acting hormonal contraceptives, forced sterilisations and abortions: the global pro-natal vs anti-national ideology at play (see Klein, 2008 and 2013).

'old eggs', 'diseased tubes'. Think of the increasing medicalisation of birth and telling women we can't make babies without doctors' advice; consider insulting terms like 'elderly primagravidas' and 'habitual aborters'. Think about the thousands of unnecessary Caesarian sections.

This is added to by the belittling and/or making illegal of midwifery as 'dangerous' and, in earlier times, the burning of witches who were midwives and healers. Then there is the *disgust* – or punishment – directed at women's monthly shedding of blood which is a sign of our fertility. This can result in religious exclusions or, like in Australia, in 2017 still having to pay a 10% Goods and Services Tax (GST) on sanitary products. As if these were 'luxury' items, when half the population needs them every month! The ongoing punishments of mothers when it comes to paid work and 'careers', and their unpaid work at home (most men still don't do half of the house work), have been the topic of many feminist books over the last 50 years, without much improvement to report. Equally, the ongoing stigmatisation of women who cannot have children – which is why the fertility industry exists – is despicable.

The 20th century has seen a constant stream of attempts to reduce women's power to reproduce life even further by creating the ultimate feat: an artificial womb. Gena Corea's powerful book *The Mother Machine* (1985) includes many examples of attempts since the 1950s to create such artificial vessels into which developing foetuses could be put (see pp. 250–259). Below are more recent examples of how some scientists continue to dream about a future when patriarchy controls which 'womb' in which part of the world is selected to have children, how many, and of what 'quality'. Grand-scale eugenics.

Utilitarian philosopher Peter Singer (who has been known to support surrogacy since the 1980s) has always been in favour of artificial wombs. In *The Reproduction Revolution: New Ways of Making Babies,* he and Deane Wells wrote in 1984 that artificial wombs would reduce the number of abortions: involuntary pregnant women could put their foetuses into this container and, when the baby was ready to be lifted out, it could be given up for adoption to infertile couples. Simple. And the topic does not go away. In 1995, liberal US feminist living in Australia, and one of Singer's acolytes, followed suit with 'Women, Ectogenesis and Ethical Theory' (Cannold, 1995).

It is a bit more surprising (but probably should not be) that in 2015, liberal feminist Evie Kendal devotes a whole book to this topic: *Equal Opportunity and the Case for State Sponsored Ectogenesis* (Kendal, 2015). She argues that an artificial womb would release women from the unfair burden (i.e. not shared with men) of having to grow a pregnancy in their bodies and give birth to a child. But how, exactly, will the 'unfair' burden stop when the child will be lifted out of its artificial container? As far as I know not even the wildest dreamers of the 'glory' that this technology will bring 'mankind' are envisaging a child to burst out of the artificial womb, ready to go to school!

So the research goes on. In 1988, Carlo Bulletti and his colleagues produced what was reported as the first case of ectogenesis in the respected US journal *Fertility and Sterility*, 'Early human pregnancy in vitro utilizing an artificially perfused uterus' (Bulletti *et al.*, 1988, pp. 991–996). The womb was not the envisaged plastic container, but the excised *live womb* of a cancer patient after a hysterectomy into which a 'spare' IVF embryo was inserted. This womb was connected to a so-called perfusion machine which, simulating the placenta, provided the embryo with oxygen, nutrients and hormones (and removed waste products) to simulate an early pregnancy. Bulletti *et al.* reported that the embryo developed 'normally' up to 52 hours. The experiment took place at the Reproductive Medicine Unit at the Department of Obstetrics and Gynecology at the University of Bologna and had, so the authors reported, been approved by the Ethical Review Board.[99]

Although this paper created international outrage, and got Bulletti sacked from his university job, he continued with his research into the artificial womb. In 2011, still in Italy, now at the Physiopathology of Reproduction Unit at Cervesi's General Hospital in Cattolica, he and Italian and French colleagues published a review article 'The artificial womb' in the *Annals of the New York Academy of Sciences* – not exactly a marginal publication (Bulletti *et al.* 2011, pp. 124–128).

---

99 I wish I could reproduce the colour images from this event that the Swiss *Tages Anzeiger Magazin* published in 1988. One shows the womb lying on the middle of the table with the perfusion tubes attached on both sides. It is bathed in the yellow glow from an overhanging light. The other image, even more chilling, is that of a gowned and masked scientist holding the womb in his hand and inserting the embryo with a syringe. I keep these images on my desk top and look at them from time to time when I need reassurance that my feminist colleagues and I are not mad: the patriarchal threat to women's existence is real and it won't stop.

As was to be expected, using the language of 'Foreground' news, Bulletti *et al.* suggest that an artificial womb – and this time they are not talking about a real woman's womb, but a container – will be useful to keep premature babies alive. Nevertheless, they also write: "Once perfected, however, an artificial womb would allow for the possibility to continue *or initiate* fetal development outside of the mother's body" (p. 125, my emphasis). So the dream of ectogenesis remains alive.

In 1996, Yoshinori Kuwabara, a gynaecologist at Tokyo University's medical department and his team, removed a 120 day-old goat foetus from its mother by Caesarean section. (120 days is about three quarters of a goat's full term pregnancy.) It was placed into a rubber womb filled with amniotic fluid. Because the artificial womb was too large, and the goat foetus kept moving too much, the researchers administered sedatives. The goat kid, which lived for a bit more than a month after it was 'born' from the container, kept suffering from the after-effects of the sedatives and could neither stand or breathe by itself (Klass, 1996; Hadfield, 1996). Nevertheless, commenting on this cruel 'achievement', Arthur L. Caplan, Director of the Center for Bioethics at the University of Pennsylvania, was excited. "Sixty years down the line ... the total artificial womb will be here. It's technologically inevitable. Demand is hard to predict, but I'll say significant" (in Klass, 1996).

So by 2056, might surrogacy be superseded by artificial wombs? With many models readily available on the internet (if that still exists) to be shipped as DIY items to (rich) households around the world? I cannot share Arthur Caplan's excitement and in my view, a pregnant woman's body, her brain, heartbeat and breath (not to mention her soul) provides a bit more than just a container to which tubes are attached. (And I don't believe the intriguing human placenta has shared all her secrets.)

But, such views – especially when expressed by respected bioethicists such as Caplan – as well as ongoing research into ectogenesis, continue the slippery slope of softening up the public who today might still have some reluctance to embrace an artificial womb. What it also does, importantly, is to *normalise* the currently available 'womb practice' with real live 'surrogate' women. What's the big deal with surrogacy when we are already considering plastic containers for breeding children?

Still, we had to wait almost twenty years until 2017 when, this time sheep mothers were sacrificed on the scientific altar. Inventing the 'Biobag', six lamb foetuses (120 to 125 days old) spent the rest of their 'pregnancy' sealed in a plastic bag (the others succumbed to sepsis or did not survive the mother's Caesarian section; she was killed after that). One lamb continued to live a seemingly normal life for over a year at the time the research was made public (25 April 2017 in *Nature Communications*; Partridge *et al.*). This time the researchers, working at the Children's Hospital at the US Philadelphia Research Institute, were careful to announce their achievement as 'An extra-uterine system to physiologically support the extreme premature lamb', thus not mentioning the 'E-word'. They state that the aim of their research is to better support prematurely born babies at 24 weeks and that first trials with human babies might begin in two years.[100]

As the US Food and Drug Administration (FDA) is reportedly fast-tracking research by Partridge *et al.* (in Spooner, 2017), we might not have to wait another twenty years for further 'exciting' news from the world of breeding babies in bags. We must also not forget that with the help of the hundreds and thousands of stockpiled 'surplus' IVF embryos that have been 'donated' to science since the 1980s, 'Background' research continues unnoticed by the general public in many laboratories around the world. And under the guise of improving the (lousy) IVF success rates, every woman undergoing IVF treatment unwittingly contributes to these endeavours when she agrees to experimental 'add-ons' such as 'assisted hatching', 'embryo glue', 'treatment for high Natural Killer Cells', testosterone 'treatments', DHEA supplementation, etc. that all cost extra money.[101]

---

100 *The Sydney Morning Herald* article by Rania Spooner (25 March 2017) contains a revealing video, showing human premature babies' suffering and authors Emily Partridge and colleagues offering hope that their 'Biobag-Breakthrough' will make premature babies' lives better; <http://www.smh.com.au/national/health/science-of-the-lambs-researchers-perfect-artificial-womb-that-works-as-well-as-ewe-do-20170425-gvrw5v.html>

101 These add-on treatments are mentioned in Julia Leigh's frank memoir *Avalanche* (2016). Two years, two Intrauterine Inseminations (IUI) and six ICSI IVF treatments later, there is no pregnancy, let alone a child. (ICSI stands for Intracytoplasmic Sperm Injection in which a single sperm is directly injected into an egg cell.) *Avalanche* describes the tens of thousands of dollars 42-year-old Julia Leigh spent on these fertility treatments, the bruising and battering of the hormonal assaults on her body which, at the end, leaves her with an ovary that is twice the normal size. Above all,

More genetic testing prior to a woman even becoming pregnant reveals more diseases, such as mitochondrial disease which is said to occur in 1 in 10,000 children and leads to early death. Once diagnosed with this disease, people wanting to have children are told that IVF with (expensive) preimplantation genetic diagnosis (PGD) is unavoidable. In December 2016, the UK Human Fertilisation and Embryology Authority (HFEA) gave the green light to 'three-person babies' allowing the use of mitochondrial replacement therapy (MRT). In MRT, the defective mitochondria in a woman's egg cell are replaced with healthy mitochondria from a 'donor' egg. (Strictly speaking, the child is a two-women, one-man baby.) This technology is controversial as it affects all cells in the future child, and will be passed on to his or her children. It is not known if it is effective, let alone safe. A boy born in Mexico after the use of MRT is not old enough to prove either (Sample, 15 December 2016). Or take Fragile X syndrome leading to intellectual and learning disabilities in the children, and Parkinson-like symptoms in

---

she shows honestly how the rollercoaster that is IVF takes over and narrows the world down to that one goal: getting pregnant. It also shows how easy it is to get 'hooked': determined to stop after the last treatment, Leigh comes precariously close to follow her IVF doctor's advice to try one more time. Luckily she does not and also makes the decision that she does not want to use 'donor' eggs or a 'surrogate'. An infuriating and heartbreaking 'must read' for any woman considering IVF. As Leigh writes (p. 44): "I had the dread feeling that I was voluntarily participating in 'cutting edge' medicine, that I was part of some greater experiment, a credulous and desperate older woman ..." Only after she has decided to stop, she asks her doctor how many 44-year old women had taken a baby home from her clinic in the last year. The answer: 2.8%.

the carrier(s). If identified in a DNA test, IVF with PGD is the next step.

There is hardly a day when we don't get news of a rare genetic disorder and see pictures of intolerable suffering. Women considering getting pregnant are then advised to seek yet another (expensive) screening test. And if they have a 'bad' gene(s), it's off to IVF. This accelerating trend is amounting to *the exploitation of fear*; the assumption that a pregnancy without medical *pre*-intervention, as well as screening *during* the baby's gestation, cannot possibly result in a healthy child (Klein, 2018). This fear mongering lets people forget that most illnesses and accidents happen after birth, and that, after all, not everything in life is predictable and screenable. It makes life so much harder for people living with disabilities for they are now blamed for their very existence ("why wasn't 'this' picked up in a test?").

But the world of reprogenetics is always inventing new tools, always moving forward and always making more money. In typical 'Foreground' hype, since the 1980s when gene therapy began to be discussed and then applied, in 2017, we are yet again told that scientists are close to eliminating horrible inherited diseases. Cystic fibrosis was a prime candidate in the 1980s; Cystic fibrosis is a prime candidate now (as was, and is, Huntington's disease and Alzheimer's). And indeed, over the last ten years, a new genetic engineering technique has become increasingly popular. It is the gene editing tool CRISPR–Cas9[102]

---

102 CRISPR stands for 'clustered regularly interspaced short palindromic repeats'. It is a guide molecule made of RNA; Cas9 is a bacterial enzyme. The CRISPR RNA is attached to Cas9 which works as molecular scissors.

that can do gene 'knockouts' or 'knockins'.[103] Put differently, CRISPR–Cas9 is a fast and inexpensive technology that can exchange single genes or whole DNA sequences with a scissor-like cut-and-paste action in plants, animals and humans.

Because CRISPR can be used for *germline* therapy in humans (i.e. exchanging genes in eggs, sperm and early embryos which will then be passed on to all future generations), the International Summit on Human Gene Editing, convened on 1–3 December 2015, issued a statement that urged caution on human germline editing, arguing that it poses many unknown dangers including the risks of inaccurate and incomplete editing of all cells and

> difficulties of predicting harmful effects ... the fact that, once introduced into the human population, genetic alterations would be difficult to remove ... the possibility that permanent genetic 'enhancements' ... could exacerbate social inequalities or be used coercively (Olson, 2015, p. 9).

Only one Summit participant – Hille Haker from Loyola University in Chicago – asked for a two-year moratorium "until an international ban on germline editing for reproductive purposes can be secured through the United Nations" (p. 5). Unfortunately, she was overruled. Germline gene therapy by any method is already a criminal offence in 29 countries – but not in the USA.

---

103 Described in this way by CRISPR–Cas9 product supplier Clontech/TaKaRa; it means that one gene or whole gene sequences can be cut out and replaced with one that does not contain the faulty gene; <http://www.clontech.com/ US/Products/Genome_Editing/CRISPR_Cas9/Resources/About_CRISPR_ Cas9>

Sure enough, we did not have to wait long to see this headline splashed across our screens on 29 July 2017: "Scientists successfully edit DNA of human embryo for first time." Vivek Wadhwa, Professor at Carnegie Mellon University Engineering at Silicon Valley, was referring to a joint US/Korean research project carried out at Oregon Health and Science University in the USA. The DNA of 131 human embryos had been edited with CRISPR-Cas9 with the aim of eliminating an inheritable heart condition (HCM) known for causing sudden death in young adults. From these in vitro manufactured human embryos – created from healthy 'donor' eggs that were injected with sperm from men suffering from this disease via IVF ICSI technology – 88% of those that developed to 4–8 cell stage embryos (blastomeres) were deemed 'successful', while 12% were not.

While a success rate of 88% is nowhere near a perfect result, it was deemed 'better' than data from previous gene edited embryos in China (in 2015 and 2016). As Wadhwa put it: "CRISPR's seductiveness is beginning to overtake the calls for caution" (29 July 2017). He also added his worries: "A former NASA fellow in synthetic biology now sells functional bacterial engineering CRISPR kits for $150 from his online store. It's not hard to imagine a future in which the big drugstores chains carry CRISPR kits for home testing and genetic engineering."

Such thoughts conjure up earlier worries from the 1980s, when gene therapy was about to take off. In 1987, noted molecular biologist and Jewish holocaust survivor, Erwin Chargaff, commenting on the advent of test-tube babies and genetic engineering, warned in *Nature* ('Engineering a Molecular

Nightmare') that, "The demand [for the technologies] was less overwhelming than the desire on the part of the scientists to test their newly developed techniques. The experimental babies produced were more of a byproduct." He further predicted the unleashing of "a molecular Auschwitz, where valuable enzymes, hormones and so on will be extracted instead of gold teeth ... we can already see the beginning of human husbandry, of industrial breeding factories" (1987, pp. 199–200). Thirty years later, we can now add our worries about the latest germline editing tool, CRISPR.

No doubt we have entered the global race of CRISPR embryo gene editing and we will see research teams compete internationally, as well as thousands of languishing 'old' gene therapy, stem cell research and cloning firms now looking forward to being revitalised, as they wait to cash in from this latest technological feat. In fact, two of the authors of the Oregon study disclose that they are shareholders and co-founders of the South Korean company ToolGen (Jin-Soo Kim, founded in 1999), and Mitogenome Therapeutics, Oregon, which Shoukhrat Mitalipov founded in 2013. (Mitalipov is also credited with being the 'father' of three-parent babies and is its intellectual property holder.)

Only time will tell if 'CRISPERing' will follow the 1990s excitement about gene therapy experiments that came to a sudden halt in 1999 when 18-year old Jesse Gelsinger died.[104]

---

104 The current hype about CRISPR is similar to the aggressive publicity in the 1980s when recombinant DNA technology (also using 'glue' and 'scissors') produced a plethora of GM bacteria and viruses. They were supposed

Or, if this time around, the new CRISPR technology will bring 'success', ultimately perhaps with genetically 'enhanced' GM children that the rich can buy. But also, potentially, with a myriad of new diseases introduced through 'faults' in the gene editing process, and problems with predicting harmful effects that genetic changes in interaction with the environment and

to create the 'Gene Revolution' and compensate for the failed 'Green Revolution' in the so-called Third World. A plethora of transgenic animals were created for the sole purpose to serve as living laboratories to test drugs for humans. It was a sad day on 13 April 1988 when Harvard University received a US patent for creating the Oncomouse: a genetically modified mouse that was highly susceptible to breast cancer which she passed on to all her offspring (Klein, 1989b, p. 258). Gene therapy experiments in humans began in 1989. Enthusiasm ran high during the 1990s without any real breakthroughs, but plenty of new global Biotech start ups, all wanting to make money. Then on 17 September 1999, 18-year old Jesse Gelsinger died in Pennsylvania. He suffered from OTCD, a metabolic disorder that affects 1 in 40,000 newborns. Gelsinger died 4 days after receiving an infusion of corrective OTC gene. His death sent shock waves through the biotechnology world and temporarily stopped gene therapy in the US (Sibbald 2001). As a Hastings Center report comments ten years after Gelsinger's death (Obasogie, 2009):

> Gene therapy was the embryonic stem cell research of the 1990s; its ability to cure was thought to be boundless and the hype was astronomical. Its promise was both therapeutic and financial: billions of dollars stood to be made from curing diseases as rare as OTCD and as common as cancer, leading several companies to invest millions in the technology.

Although human gene therapy trials resumed, more deaths and mishaps occurred, such as an American woman's death in 2008 after an injection with an experimental arthritis gene. This followed an earlier setback in 2002 when leukemia developed after the insertion of a retrovirus in a gene therapy trial for X-linked severe combined immunodeficiency (Evans *et al.*, 2008). We can only hope that the use of CRISPR will not result in similar tragedies.

other living organisms might produce. We have, of course, seen this already happening with plant and animal GM technologies for decades and it has led to many failures and 'genetic roulette' (see Hawthorne, 2002, pp. 242–248 and Robin, 2010, pp. 149–152).

At any rate, for any chance of CRISPR fulfilling its potential role to edit human germline cells and early embryos, *thousands* of young women will be required to produce healthy egg cells by undergoing the dangerous egg maturation and extraction procedures described in Chapter 2 (pp. 13–15 and pp. 20–21). And once the genes of in vitro manufactured early embryos have been 'edited' with 'knockouts' and knockins', some rogue scientist(s) somewhere in the world 'playing God' will want to implant them in real live women to see what 'capability enhanced' babies they can create. (Unless, of course, the *human* Biobag has been perfected.[105])

---

105 Or eggs and sperm cells might be produced in unlimited numbers from human skin cells in a process called IVG (in vitro gametogenesis, as reported on 12 January, 2017 and so far only achieved in mice; Sample, 2017). With all these gametes available in the lab, unlimited numbers of embryos could be created. This 'egg heaven' (sperm has always been easy to get) would no doubt make reprogenetic researchers very happy. For decades they have complained about the dearth of egg cells: "I would have been content if only human eggs had come my way more freely" lamented Robert Edwards in 1980 when he talked about "dreaming of eggs" and the many frustrations before the birth of Louise Brown in 1978 when he had to use cow eggs for his experiments (in Corea, 1984, p. 42). In 1987, it looked as if the limitless egg dreams might be fulfilled soon when immature eggs, taken from cow ovaries, were matured in vitro and turned into 'test-tube' calves (Vines, 1987, p. 23). The next idea was to cut out a wedge from a *woman's* ovary with hundreds of immature egg cells and mature them in the lab (women have

When Andrea Dworkin and Gena Corea predicted in the 1980s that so-called surrogates might be kept in 'reproductive brothels' in third world countries, they were laughed at and chided for their scaremongering. But their predictions came true. What will stop the next wave of poor women in unregulated countries being implanted with CRISPR embryos – unless CRISPR too turns out to be a failure like earlier gene therapy techniques.

This is where the CRISPR excursion leads us straight back to the egg 'donor' and surrogacy story that I have told in this book. I believe it is crucially important that we keep an eye on 'Background' events such as new biotechnological developments. If the CRISPR craze continues, thousands of healthy human eggs will be needed, which means thousands of egg 'donors' may be harmed. Similarly, the 'Background' *and* 'Foreground' trend to screen for a skyrocketing number of rare genetic diseases will increase the number of women that are referred to IVF programs, undergo egg maturation/collection

---

about 400,000 egg cells in our ovaries of which only 350 to 400 ripen in a life time; Klein 1989b, p. 275). In 1988, the 'egg fever' reached Australia and in 'Foreground' speak, we were told by IVF doctors that limitless access to egg cells would greatly increase IVF success rates. But it was Max Brinsmead, a reproductive physiologist at the University of Newcastle who had the media go wild when he suggested that harvesting immature egg cells from the ovaries in foetuses might be a great idea: "A foetus which is not even born could ultimately have children ... by the 14th week it contains its full complement of 100 million oocytes. ... Terminated foetuses or non-surviving neonates could theoretically become egg donors" (in Miller, 1988). To my knowledge this lunacy was never attempted; if it had, we might be closer to Brave New World today. We'll have to wait and see if IVG fulfils the scientists' egg wish, or if it too drops off the cliff, as so many of these technologies do.

and then have their embryo(s) screened with preimplantation genetic diagnosis (PGD). When these pregnancies fail (as they did for Julia Leigh in *Avalanche*), the next step is likely to be surrogacy. So the number of 'surrogate' mothers required will increase, as will the number of tests they then have to submit to, including PGD, by the forewarned 'commissioning parents'.

So, what can we do? First and foremost, I suggest we need a serious and worldwide public discussion about the many problems and dangers that surrogacy entails. Call me naïve but I stubbornly continue to believe that most people including those fervently wishing for their own genetically related child, are decent human beings who would not knowingly want to violate the human rights of the women involved in surrogacy or indeed those of the resulting children.

We need to break through the 'hype' and happy stories that pro-surrogacy advocacy groups, IVF clinics and the (social) media unleash on us. We have to understand that not supporting gay men when they claim to have a 'right' to exploit two women so they can have 'their' baby, is not homophobia. We need to find other gay men like Gary Powell and Raul Solis from the UK and Spain to speak out against surrogacy. In Australia, two of the most prominent supporters of surrogacy are openly gay men; we need other gay men to come forward and engage the LGBTI community so they understand the fundamental problems with surrogacy and do not end up splitting these groups as most lesbians neither need nor support surrogacy.

Many gay men, and many heterosexual men with fertility problems can, and do, make great parents, be it in foster care or permanent care arrangements (which is better for the child than adoption, see Mackieson, 2015). Or, quite simply in making a commitment to regularly spending time with the children of their friends or siblings, and supporting them through the 'fun' as well as the hard times. And there are many jobs that require dedicated child-centred professionals. Ask yourself if your desire for children is about the *joy* of spending time with children, or if it is about possession: wanting to *own* a child that you have bought (or at least solicited).

Surrogacy has to stop being seen as 'cool' in the same way that young men in countries with so-called Nordic Laws which criminalise sex buyers have stopped buying prostituted women; they perceive it as unethical. We also, yet again, need another discussion like the one we had in the 1980s and 1990s that a 'child-free' life is not a second-class and/or egotistical life, but a life that offers many rewards and does not mean that you 'hate' children and have no children in your life (see Rowland, 1992, pp. 251–256). For that to happen, many antiquated prejudices about the 'roles' of women as 'childbearers' and men as 'bread-winners' that continue to persist against all odds, need to be finally put to rest.

We must not forget that for those of us living a middle-class life in westernised states (or as part of the 'elite' of a poor country), pro-natalist ideology has never gone away. This 'motherhood imperative' causes society and women with a fertility problem to see themselves as 'deficient' and 'abnormal'. This sense of failure is precisely what IVF clinics exploit with their baby-bliss advertising in order to suck women onto expensive IVF treatment mills. If you are an Indigenous woman and/or part of a non-mainstream ethnic, poor group, and/or living with a disability in a westernised country (or indeed, a non-elite citizen of a poor country), IVF is not for you. Instead you get the hormonal cocktails, implants or needles for the anti-natalist 'prevention of pregnancy'. As for surrogacy, I have never heard of a poor woman anywhere in the world engaging in surrogacy as a 'buyer'; she is always the 'seller' with all the problems and dangers this entails.

Apart from demystifying what really goes on in surrogacy, I would also like governments in countries such as Australia, that may be tempted to think about devising model laws for 'best practice' 'altruistic' surrogacy, to rethink the idea that 'regulation' can ever be the answer. It can not and in fact, as I have argued in Chapter 5, regulation will only ever *cement* surrogacy as 'legitimate'. And it will enshrine the compartmentalisation of women reduced to body parts, and encourage dissociative mechanisms to cope with the inherent cruelty. We also do well to remember that *any* regulation will be subverted by those who do not want to abide by its laws. Much better for a government to invest in a funded public education campaign that goes to the *root* of what surrogacy is: a deeply unethical practice that exploits and commodifies 'surrogate' mothers, egg 'donors', and their birth children.

Most importantly, we must never shrug our shoulders and say "oh well, surrogacy exists, let's just regulate it and make it ethical." Women and their children who get harmed in the surrogacy industry deserve better. Neoliberals (feminists included) have to seriously consider whether they want to continue to support the surrogacy industry when it breaks about every existing UN convention and other international agreements. Moreover, as I have described in Chapter 6, we now have a fantastic model that we can support and work with: The International Convention for the Abolition of Surrogacy (see pp. 99–102).

I know there are many like-minded individuals around the globe and I appeal to your sense of fairness to join us and do your utmost to stop this dehumanising trade that creates children who are 'for sale'. The multi-billion capitalist and patriarchal surrogacy business exploits women everywhere in the world on the basis of class, race and ethnicity and, because of its inbuilt eugenic practices, works against the interests of people with disabilities. Women living in poverty are particularly badly exploited.

As I have emphasised throughout this book, the whole surrogacy industry is so deeply problematic on so many fronts, that it is hard to understand why anyone with a social justice conscience could support it.

Please join our campaign to Stop Surrogacy Now.

Bibliography

ABC Television (12 July 2007). 'The 7.30 Report with Kerry O'Brien'. Australian Broadcasting Company, Sydney.

ABC Television (22 September 2014). 'Made in Thailand'. *Four Corners*. Reporters Debbie Whitmont and Karen Michelmore; <http://www.abc.net.au/4corners/stories/2014/09/22/4090232.htm>

ABC News (11 August 2014). 'Searching for C11 – Transcript'. *Australian Story*; <http://www.abc.net.au/austory/content/2014/s4065081.htm>

ABC News (21 August 2014). 'What chance for international surrogacy laws?'; <http://www.abc.net.au/news/2014-08-21/van-whichelen-what-chance-for-international-surrogacy-laws/5683746>

ABC News (29 June 2017). 'Baby Gammy is Now Three'; <http://www.abc.net.au/news/2017-06-29/baby-gammy-is-now-three/8662868>

Achtelik, Kirsten (2015). *Selbstbestimmte Norm. Feminismus, Pränataldiagnostik, Abtreibung*. Verbrecher Verlag, Berlin.

Akhter, Farida, Wilma Van Berkel and Natasha Ahmed (eds.) (1989). *The Comilla Declaration*. FINRRAGE/UBINIG Proceedings. Dhaka.

Akhter, Farida (1992). *Depopulating Bangladesh: Essays on the Politics of Fertility*. Narigrantha Prabartana, Dhaka.

Akhter, Farida (1995). *Resisting Norplant*. Narigrantha Prabartana, Dhaka.

Allan, Sonia (5 August 2014). 'Gammy case highlights risks of for-profit surrogacy market'. *The Sydney Morning Herald*; <http://www.smh.com.au/comment/gammy-case-highlights-risks-of-forprofit-surrogacy-market-20140803-1003fr.html>

Allan, Sonia (2016). 'Submission No. 17 to the Inquiry into the Regulatory and Legislative Aspects of International and Domestic Surrogacy Arrangements, House of Representatives Standing Committee on Social Policy and Legal Affairs, Parliament of Australia';

<http://www.aph.gov.au/Parliamentary_Business/Committees/House/Social_Policy_and_Legal_Affairs/Inquiry_into_surrogacy/Submissions>

Arditti, Rita, Renate Duelli Klein and Shelley Minden (eds.) (1984/1989). *Test-tube Women: What Future for Motherhood?* Pandora Press, London; Allen and Unwin, Sydney.

Arditti, Rita (1988). 'A Summary of some recent developments on surrogacy in the United States' *Reproductive and Genetic Engineering* Vol. 1, No. 1, pp. 51–64.

Atwood, Margaret (1985). *The Handmaid's Tale*. McClelland and Stewart, Toronto.

Bachinger, Eva Maria (2015). *Kind auf Bestellung*. Deuticke im Paul Zsolnay Verlag, Vienna.

Barker, Anne (23 February 2017). 'Desperate Australian couples unable to leave Cambodia with surrogate babies'; <http://www.abc.net.au/news/2017-02-23/australian-couples-with-surrogate-babies-stuck-in-cambodia/8294810>

Barker, Anne (21 November, 2016). 'Australian woman charged with running illegal surrogacy clinics in Cambodia'; <http://www.abc.net.au/news/2016-11-21/australian-woman-charged-over-illegal-surrogacy-clinic-cambodia/8042708>

BBC News (7 August 2014). 'Thai surrogate baby Gammy: Australian parents contacted'; <http://www.bbc.com/news/world-asia-28686114>

Beekman, Madeleine (20 November 2015). 'Do you share more genes with your mother or your father?' *The Conversation*; <http://theconversation.com/do-you-share-more-genes-with-your-mother-or-your-father-50076?utm_medium=email&utm_campaign=The+Weekend+Conversation+-+3848&utm_content=The+Weekend+Conversation+-+3848+CID_61a7cc1a201fc294d7e8dd96475391da&utm_source=campaign_monitor&utm_term=Do%20you%20share%20more%20genes%20with%20your%20mother%20or%20your%20father>

Bell, Diane and Renate Klein (eds.) (1996). *Radically Speaking: Feminism Reclaimed*. Spinifex Press, North Melbourne.

Bindel, Julie (2017). *The Pimping of Prostitution: Abolishing the Sex Work Myth*. Palgrave Macmillan, London; Spinifex Press, Geelong and Mission Beach.

Bradish, Paula, Erika Feyerabend and Ute Winkler (eds.) (1989). *Frauen gegen Gen- und Reproduktionstechnologien*. Frauenoffensive, München.

Brennan, Bridget (18 April 2015). 'Surrogacy reform needed to encourage "ethical" arrangements: Chief Justice'. *ABC AM*; <http://www.abc.net.au/news/2015-04-18/surrogacy-reform-needed-to-encourage-ethical/6402844>

Brodribb, Somer (1992). *Nothing Mat(t)ers*. Spinifex Press, North Melbourne.

Bulletti, Carlo, Valerio M Jasonni, Stefania Tabanelli, Lucca Gianaroli, Patrizia M Ciotti, Anna P Ferraretti and Carlo Flamigni (June 1988). 'Early human pregnancy *in vitro* utilizing an artificially perfused uterus'. *Fertility and Sterility*, Vol. 49, Issue 6, pp. 991–996.

Bulletti, Carlo, Antonio Palagiano, Caterina Pace, Angelica Cerni, Andrea Borini and Dominique de Ziegler (2011). 'The Artificial Womb'. *Annals of the New York Academy of Science*, Vol. 1221, pp. 124–128.

Canberra Times (20 October 1988). 'IVF Triplets' Surrogate Birth in Perth'; <http://trove.nla.gov.au/newspaper/rendition/nla.news-article 102016161.txt?print+true>

Cannold, Leslie (1995). 'Women, Ectogenesis and Ethical Theory'. *Journal of Applied Philosophy*, Vol. 12, No. 1, pp. 55–64.

Cannold, Leslie (2006). 'Women can still say no'. *On Line Opinion*; <http://www.onlineopinion.com.au/view.asp?article=5197&page=0>

Chargaff, Erwin (1987). 'Engineering a Molecular Nightmare'. *Nature*, Vol. 327, Issue 6119, pp. 199–200.

Chesler, Phyllis (1972). *Women and Madness*. Doubleday, Garden City, New York.

Chesler, Phyllis (1987). *Mothers on Trial: The Battle for Children and Custody*. Seal Press, Seattle.

Chesler, Phyllis (1988). *Sacred Bond: The Legacy of Baby M*. Crown Publishing Group, New York.

Commonwealth of Australia (2006). 'The Prohibition of Human Cloning and the Regulation of Human Embryo Research Amendment Bill 2006'; <https://www.legislation.gov.au/Details/C2006A00172>

Corea, Gena (1984). 'Egg Snatchers' in Rita Arditti, Renate Duelli Klein and Shelley Minden (eds.) (1984/1989). *Test-tube Women: What Future for Motherhood?* Pandora Press, London; Allen and Unwin, Sydney, pp. 37–51.

Corea, Gena (1985). *The Mother Machine: Reproductive Technologies from Artificial Insemination to Artificial Wombs.* Harper and Row, New York.

Corea, Gena, Renate Duelli Klein, Jalna Hanmer, Helen B Holmes, Betty Hoskins, Madhu Kishwar *et al.* (1985/1987). *Man-made Women: How New Reproductive Technologies Affect Women.* Hutchinson, London; Indiana University Press, Bloomington.

Corea, Gena (1989). 'Mère porteuse et liberté'. In *L'ovaire-dose?* Actes du colloque organisé les 3 et 4 décembre 1988 par le MFPF (Mouvement français pour le planning familial). Catherine Lesterpt and Gatienne Doat (eds.). Syros/Alternatives, Paris, pp. 259–275.

Corea, Gena and Cynthia de Wit (1988). 'Current Developments' in *Reproductive and Genetic Engineering: Journal of International Feminist Analysis*, Vol. 1, No. 2, pp. 183–203.

CoRP (Collectif pour le Respect de la Personne), Cadac (Coordination des associations pour le droit à l'avortement et à la contraception), CLF (Coordination lesbienne en France) *et al.* (2015). 'The International Convention for the Abolition of Surrogacy': <https://collectifcorp.files.wordpress.com/2015/01/surrogacy_hcch_feminists_english.pdf>

Cotton, Kim and Denise Winn (1985). *For Love and Money.* Dorling Kindersley Publishers, London.

Creative Family Connections; <http://www.creativefamilyconnections.com/us-surrogacy-law-map>

Daly, Mary (1978). *Gyn/Ecology: The Metaethics of Radical Feminism.* Beacon Press, Boston.

Darnovsky, Marcy and Diane Beeson (December 2014). 'Global Surrogacy Practices'. Working Paper No. 601, *International Institute of Social Studies (ISS)*, The Hague, Netherlands; < https://repub.eur.nl/pub/77402>

Dawe, Gavin S, Tan, Xiao Wei, and Xiao, Zhi-Cheng (January-March 2007). 'Cell Migration from Baby to Mother'. *Cell Adhesion and Migration*, Vol. 1, No. 3.

Deccan Chronicle (3 July 2017). 'Womb transplants for men; revolution in reproduction poses moral dilemma'; <http://www.deccanchronicle. com/lifestyle/health-and-wellbeing/030717/wombs-for-men-revolution-in-reproduction-poses-moral-dilemma.html>

Derek, Julia (2004). *Confessions of a Serial Egg Donor*. Adrenaline Books, New York.

De Saille, Stevienna (2018). *Knowledge as Resistance: The Feminist International Network of Resistance to Reproductive and Genetic Engineering*. Palgrave Macmillan, London.

Die Grünen im Bundestag, AK Frauenpolitik und sozialwissenschaftliche Forschung und Praxis für Frauen (1985). 'Frauen gegen Gentechnik und Reproduktionstechnik.' Dokumentation zum Kongress vom 19–21.4.1985 in Bonn. Die Grünen, Köln.

Dworkin, Andrea (1983). *Right-Wing Women: The Politics of Domesticated Females*. The Women's Press, London.

Ekman, Kajsa Ekis (2013). *Being and Being Bought: Prostitution, Surrogacy and the Split Self*. Spinifex Press, North Melbourne.

Elenis, Evangelia, Agneta Skoog Svanberg, Alkistis Skalkidou, and Gunilla Sydsjö (8 October, 2015). 'Adverse obstetric outcomes in pregnancies resulting from oocyte donation: a retrospective cohort case study in Sweden.' *BMC Pregnancy Childbirth*, 15, 247; <https://www.ncbi.nlm. nih.gov/pmc/articles/PMC4598963/>

European Parliament (5 April 2011). 'Resolution on priorities and outline of a new EU policy framework to fight violence against women'; <http://www.europarl.europa.eu/sides/getDoc.do?pubRef=-//EP// TEXT+TA+P7-TA-2011-0127+0+DOC+XML+V0//EN>

European Parliament (16 December 2015). 'Motion on the Annual Report on Human Rights and Democracy in the World 2014 and the European Union's policy on the matter'; <http://www.europarl.europa. eu/sides/getDoc.do?pubRef=-//EP//TEXT+REPORT+A8-2015-0344+0+DOC+XML+V0//EN#title1>

Evans, Christopher H, Steven C Ghivizzani and Paul D Robbins (27 May 2008). 'Arthritis gene therapy's first death'. *Biomed Central*, Vol. 10, No. 110; <https://arthritis-research.biomedcentral.com/articles/ 10.1186/ar2411>

Everingham, Sam/Bernadette Tobin (14 May 2015). 'Should commercial surrogacy be legal in Australia?' *Sydney Morning Herald*; <http://www.smh.com.au/comment/should-commercial-surrogacy-be-legal-in-australia-20150514-gh1ead.html>

Feneley, Rick (30 April 2015). 'Chief Justice Diana Bryant confident commercial surrogacy will be legalised in Australia.' *Sydney Morning Herald*; <http://www.smh.com.au/national/chief-justice-diana-bryant-confident-commercial-surrogacy-will-be-legalised-in-australia-20150429-1mvzn1.html>

FINRRAGE/UBINIG (1989). *The Declaration of Comilla*; <http://www.finrrage.org/wpcontent/uploads/2016/03/Comilla_Proceedings_1989.pdf>

FINRRAGE (2016). 'Submission No. 70 to the Inquiry into the Regulatory and Legislative Aspects of International and Domestic Surrogacy Arrangements, House of Representatives Standing Committee on Social Policy and Legal Affairs, Parliament of Australia'; <http://www.aph.gov.au/Parliamentary_Business/Committees/House/Social_Policy_and_Legal_Affairs/Inquiry_into_surrogacy/Submissions>

Foster, Judy with Marlene Derlet (2013). *Invisible Women of Prehistory: Three Million Years of Peace, Six Thousand Years of War*. Spinifex Press, North Melbourne.

Fraser, Jo (2016). 'Submission No. 29 to the Inquiry into the Regulatory and Legislative Aspects of International and Domestic Surrogacy Arrangements, House of Representatives Standing Committee on Social Policy and Legal Affairs, Parliament of Australia'; <http://www.aph.gov.au/Parliamentary_Business/Committees/House/Social_Policy_and_Legal_Affairs/Inquiry_into_surrogacy/Submissions>

Garr, John D (2012). *Feminine by Design: The God-Fashioned Woman*. Golden Key Press, Atlanta GA.

Gillard, Julia (21 March 2013). 'National Apology for Forced Adoptions'; <https://www.youtube.com/watch?v=5hVbokTpYeg>

Goldstein, Bonnie (23 July 2009). 'In surrogacy, a deal is not always a deal.' *Slate*; <http://www.slate.com/articles/podcasts/amicus/2017/06/the_2016_supreme_court_term_in_review_on_amicus.html>

Bibliography

Gopal, M Sai (19 June 2017). 'Is Hyderabad turning into a surrogacy hub?'; <https://telanganatoday.com/is-hyderabad-turning-into-surrogacy-hub>

Gouvernment du Québec, Conseil du statut de la femme (1988). *Sortir la maternité du laboratoire*. Actes du forum international sur les nouvelles technologies de la réproduction organisé par le Conseil du statut de la femme et tenu a Montréal les 29, 30 et 31 octobre 1987 a l'Université Concordia, Canada.

Hadfield, Peter (29 September 1996). 'Japanese pioneers raise kid in rubber womb'. *New Scientist*; <https://www.newscientist.com/article/mg13418180-400-japanese-pioneers-raise-kid-in-rubber-womb/>

Hands Off Our Ovaries (2006). 'Mission Statement'; <http://www.handsoffourovaries.com/manifesto.htm?>

Hawley, Samantha (2 September 2014). 'Australian charged with sexually abusing twins he fathered with Thai surrogate'. *ABC News*; <http://www.abc.net.au/news/2014-09-01/australian-who-fathered-surrogate-twins-facing-abuse-charges/5710796>

Hawthorne, Susan (2002). *Wild Politics: Feminism, Globalisation, Bio/diversity*. Spinifex Press, North Melbourne.

Higgins, Claire (2008). *Assisted Reproductive Technology Bill 2008*. Parliament of Victoria, Melbourne; <http://trove.nla.gov.au/version/43419158>

Holmes, Helen B, Betty Hoskins and Michael Gross (eds.) (1981). *The Custom-Made Child: Women-Centered Perspectives*. The Humana Press Inc., Clifton, New Jersey.

House of Representatives Standing Committee on Social Policy and Legal Affairs (April 2016). *Surrogacy Matters: Inquiry into the Regulatory and Legislative Aspects of International and Domestic Surrogacy Arrangements*. Commonwealth of Australia, Canberra; <http://www.aph.gov.au/Parliamentary_Business/Committees/House/Social_Policy_and_Legal_Affairs/Inquiry_into_surrogacy/Report>

Humbyrd, Casey (2009). 'Fair Trade International Surrogacy'. *Developing World Bioethics*, Vol. 9, No. 3; <https://www.ncbi.nlm.nih.gov/pubmed/19508290>

Hurley, Jennifer (20 January 1989). '"Surrogate" Motherhood: Advocacy and Resistance, Linda Kirkman and Elizabeth Kane'. In *Girls Own Annual*, Deakin University, Geelong, pp. 22–23.

Ince, Susan (1984/1989). 'Inside the Surrogate Industry' in *Test-tube Women: What Future for Motherhood*? Pandora Press, London; Allen and Unwin, Sydney, pp. 99–116.

International Board for Regression Therapy (n.d.) 'Homepage'; <http://www.ibrt.orgtehead>

Jewett, Christina (2 February 2017). 'Women fear drug they used to halt puberty led to health problems'. *California Healthline;* <http://californiahealthline.org/news/women-fear-drug-they-used-to-halt-puberty-led-to-health-problems/?utm_campaign=CHL%3A+Daily+Edition&utm_source=hs_email&utm_medium=email&utm_content=41855826&_hsenc=p2ANqtz-_zWvmRa1NxYrvwMmqnhCU1R2dtqpRmA83E9-7lKoofvLctmgSgCnVnP1lqY1XDxk47IjqBUK7M37824YkdX0rMLkELRQ&_hsmi=41855826>

Kane, Elisabeth (1988/90). *Birth Mother: The Story of America's First Legal Surrogate Mother*. Harcourt, San Diego; Sun Books, Macmillan, South Melbourne (with a Foreword by Robyn Rowland).

Kaupen-Haas, Heidrun (1988). 'Experimental Obstetrics and National Socialism: The conceptual basis of reproductive technology today'. *Reproductive and Genetic Engineering: Journal of International Feminist Analysis*, Vol. 1, No. 2, pp. 127–132.

Katz Rothman, Barbara (1986). *The Tentative Pregnancy: Prenatal Diagnosis and the Future of Motherhood*. Viking Penguin, New York.

Katz Rothman, Barbara (1989). *Recreating Motherhood: Ideology and Technology in a Patriarchal Society*. W.W. Norton and Co, New York and London.

Kendal, Evie (2015). *Equal Opportunity and the Case for State Sponsored Ectogenesis*. Palgrave Macmillan, London.

Kirkman Maggie and Linda Kirkman (1988). *My Sister's Child*. Penguin, Melbourne.

Kirkman, Maggie (2002). 'Sister-to-Sister Surrogacy 13 years on: A narrative of parenthood'. *Journal of Reproduction and Infant Psychology*, Vol. 20, No. 3, pp. 135–147.

Bibliography

Klass, Perri (29 September 1996). 'The Artificial Womb is Born'. *The New York Times Magazine*; <http://www.nytimes.com/1996/09/29/magazine/the-artificial-womb-is-born.html>

Klein, Renate (1989a). *The Exploitation of a Desire: Women's Experiences with in vitro fertilisation*. Deakin University, Geelong.

Klein, Renate/Robyn Rowland (1988). 'Women as test-sites for fertility drugs. Clomiphene citrate and hormonal cocktails'. *Reproductive and Genetic Engineering* Vol. 1, No, 3, pp. 251–274.

Klein, Renate D (ed) (1989b). *Infertility: Women Speak Out about Their Experiences of Reproductive Medicine*. Pandora Press, London.

Klein, Renate, Janice G Raymond and Lynette J Dumble (1991/2013). *RU 486: Misconceptions, Myths and Morals*. Spinifex Press, North Melbourne.

Klein, Renate (1996). '(Dead) Bodies Floating in Cyberspace: Postmodernism and the Dismemberment of Women' in Diane Bell and Renate Klein (eds.) *Radically Speaking: Feminism Reclaimed*. Spinifex Press, North Melbourne, pp. 346–358.

Klein, Renate (2006). 'Rhetoric of Choice clouds dangers of harvesting women's eggs for cloning'. *On Line Opinion*; <http://www.handsoffourovaries.com/manifesto.htm>

Klein, Renate (2008). 'From Test-tube Women to Women without Bodies'. *Women's Studies International Forum* Vol. 31, pp. 157–175.

Klein, Renate (June 2011). 'Surrogacy in Australia: New Legal Developments'. *Bioethics Research Notes*, Vol. 23, No. 2, pp. 23–26; <http://www.cam.org.au/News-and-Events/News-and-Events/Melbourne-News/Article/14966/Reproductive-slavery-.Vl00q3ui1_w>

Klein, Renate (20 August 2014). 'Baby Gammy has shown the need for debate on surrogacy'. *The Sydney Morning Herald*; <http://www.smh.com.au/comment/baby-gammy-has-shown-the-need-for-debate-on-surrogacy-20140819-105pfx.html>

Klein, Renate (29 March 2015a). 'Reflections on Roundtable on Surrogacy' Standing Committee on Social Policy and Legal Affairs, March 5 2015, Parliament House, Canberra.

Klein, Renate (18 May 2015b). 'Can Surrogacy Be Ethical?'; <http://www.abc.net.au/religion/articles/2015/05/18/4237872.htm>

Klein, Renate (2018). 'The Exploitation of Fear: How Wunschkinder have to be perfect'. DFG/South Asia Institute, University of Heidelberg.

Lahl, Jennifer and Melinda Tankard Reist (eds.)(2018). *Broken Bonds: Surrogate Mothers Speak Out*. Spinifex Press, Geelong and Mission Beach.

Lahl, Jennifer (May 2016). 'Telling the Truth about Surrogacy in the United States'. The Center for Bioethics and Culture Network, Pleasant Hill, California; <http://bit.ly/2fEHTRR>

Leigh, Julia (2016). *Avalanche: A Love Story*. Hamish Hamilton, Melbourne.

Lesterpt, Catherine and Gatienne Doat (eds.) (1989). *L'ovaire-dose? : Les nouvelles methodes de procréation. Actes du colloque organisé les 3 et 4 décembre 1988 par le Mouvement français pour le planning familial*. Syros/Alternatives, Paris.

Lynch, Catherine (2016). 'Submission No. 13 on behalf of the Australian Adoptee Rights Action Group, to the Inquiry into the Regulatory and Legislative Aspects of International and Domestic Surrogacy Arrangements, House of Representatives Standing Committee on Social Policy and Legal Affairs, Parliament of Australia.'; <http://www.aph.gov.au/Parliamentary_Business/Committees/House/Social_Policy_and_Legal_Affairs/Inquiry_into_surrogacy/Submissions>

Mackieson, Penny (2015). *Adoption Deception: A Personal and Professional Journey*. Spinifex Press, North Melbourne.

Marre, Diana and Beatriz San Román (eds.) (November 2015). International Forum on Intercountry Adoption and Global Surrogacy, AFIN, No. 77, Barcelona; <https://ddd.uab.cat/pub/afin/afinENG/afin_a2015m11n77iENG.pdf>

Marsh, Beezy (3 December 2006). 'IVF can lower chance of pregnancy'. *The Telegraph* (UK).

Masoudian, PA Nasr, J de Nanassy, K Fung-Kee-Fung, SA Bainbridge and D El Demellawy (March 2016). 'Oocyte donation pregnancies and the risk of preeclampsia or gestational hypertension: a systematic review and metaanalysis'. *American Journal of Obstetrics and Gynecology*, Vol. 214, No. 3, pp. 328–39; <https://www.ncbi.nlm.nih.gov/pubmed/26627731>

Medew, Julia (23 March 2013). 'Surrogacy's painful path to parenthood'; <http://www.smh.com.au/national/surrogacys-painful-path-to-parenthood-20130322-2glhn.html>

Meggett, Marie (ed) (1991). 'Surrogacy – In Whose Interest?' Proceedings of National Conference on Surrogacy. Mission of St James and St John, West Melbourne.

Mies, Maria (1985). 'Why Do We Need All This? A Call Against Genetic Engineering and Reproductive Technology'. *Women's Studies International Forum* Vol. 8, No. 6, pp. 553–560.

Mies, Maria (1986). *Patriarchy and Accumulation on a World Scale: Women in the International Division of Labour.* Zed Books, London; Spinifex Press, North Melbourne.

Mies, Maria (1988). 'Selbstbestimmung – das Ende einer Utopie?' in Paula Bradish, Erika Feyerabend and Ute Winkler (eds.) (1989). *Frauen gegen Gen- und Reproduktionstechnologien.* Frauenoffensive, München, pp. 111–124.

Miller, Calvin (27 May 1988). 'When a foetus is a mother'. *Australian Doctor.*

Millican, Lynne (May 2, 2014). 'Hidden Clinical Trial Data About Lupron'. *Impact Ethics;* <https://impactethics.ca/2014/05/02/hidden-clinical-trial-data-about-lupron/>

Millican, Lynne (2017); <lupronvictimshub/lawsuits.html>

Monks, John (15 September 1989). 'I'll have your Surrogate Baby'. *New Idea*, pp. 12–13.

Morgan, Robin (1989/2001). *Demon Lover: The Roots of Terrorism.* W.W. Norton and Co., New York; Washington Square Press/Simon and Schuster, New York.

Munro, Kathryn (1997). 'Technogyny: The Transformation of Reproduction'. PhD Thesis, Deakin University, Victoria.

Murdoch, Lindsay (20 November 2016). 'Australian nurse Tammy Davis-Charles arrested in Cambodian surrogacy crackdown'. *The Sydney Morning Herald;* <http://www.smh.com.au/world/australian-nurse-tammy-charles-caught-up-in-cambodian-surrogacy-crackdown-20161120-gstd23.html>

Nicolau, Yona, Austin Purkeypile, T Allen Merritt, Mitchell Goldstein and Bryan Oshiro (10 November 2015). 'Outcomes of surrogate pregnancies in California and hospital economics of surrogate maternity and newborn care'. *World Journal of Obstetrics and Gynecology*, Vol. 4, Issue 4, pp. 1–6.

Norma, Caroline and Tankard Reist, Melinda (2016). *Prostitution Narratives: Stories of Survival in the Sex Trade.* Spinifex Press, North Melbourne.

Norris, Sonya and Marlisa Tiedemann (1911). 'Legal Status at the Federal Level of Assisted Human Reproduction in Canada'; <https://lop.parl.ca/Content/LOP/ResearchPublications/2011-82-e.htm?cat=government:>

Obasogie, Osagie K (22 October 2009). 'Ten Years Later: Jesse Gelsinger's Death and Human Subject Protection'. *The Hastings Center*; <http://www.thehastingscenter.org/ten-years-later-jesse-gelsingers-death-and-human-subjects-protection/>

Olson, Stephen (December 2015). 'International Summit on Human Gene Editing: A Global Discussion'; <https://www.ncbi.nlm.nih.gov/books/NBK343651/>

Page, Stephen (18 December 2016). 'Family Court of Australia court registers US pre-birth surrogacy order'; <http://surrogacyandadoption.blogspot.com.au/search?updated-max=2017-01-29T15:34:00%2B10:00&max-results=7&start=21&by-date=false>

Pande, Amrita (2014). *Wombs in Labor: Transnational Commercial Surrogacy in India.* Columbia University Press, New York.

Pande, Amrita (2015). 'Global Reproductive Inequalities, Neo-Eugenics and Commercial Surrogacy in India'. *Current Sociology*, pp. 1–15.

Pande, Amrita (29 August, 2016). 'Surrogates are Workers, not Wombs'. *The Hindu*; <http://www.thehindu.com/opinion/op-ed/Surrogates-are-workers-not-wombs/article14594820.ece>

Pande, Amrita (2017). 'Transnational commercial surrogacy in India: to ban or not to ban'. In Miranda Davies (ed) *Babies for Sale? Transnational Surrogacy, Human Rights and the Politics of Reproduction*, Zed Books, London, pp. 328–343.

Partridge, Emily A, Marcus G Davey, Matthew A Hornick *et al.* (25 April 2017). 'An extra-uterine system to physiologically support the extreme premature lamb'. *Nature Communications*; <http://www.nature.com/articles/ncomms15112>

Pearlman, Jonathan (30 May 2017). 'Australia unveils new plan to confiscate paedophiles' passports in bid to crack down on predatory tourism'. *The Telegraph*; <http://www.telegraph.co.uk/news/2017/05/30/australia-unveils-new-plan-confiscate-paedophiles-passports/>

Powell, Gary (2015). 'Why I Support #StopSurrogacyNow'; <http://www.stopsurrogacynow.com/why-i-support-stopsurrogacynow/#sthash.qx9MuHns.dpbs>

Radio National (2014). 'e-Baby: the surrogate story'; <http://www.abc.net.au/radionational/programs/drawingroom/e-baby/6273604>

Rajan, Sanoj (January 2017). 'International surrogacy arrangements and statelessness' in *The World's Stateless Children*. Institute on Statelessness and Inclusion/Wolf Legal Publishers, Oisterwijk, The Netherlands, pp. 374–384; <http://www.institutesi.org/worldsstateless17.pdf>

Ralston, Nick (30 June 2013). 'Named: the Australian paedophile jailed for 40 years', *Sydney Morning Herald*; <http://www.smh.com.au/national/named-the-australian-paedophile-jailed-for-40-years-20130630-2p5da.html>

Rao, Mohan (September 2016). 'Banning commercial surrogacy is the only way forward'. *GovernanceNow* pp. 38–39.

Raymond, Janice G (1986/2001). *A Passion for Friends: Toward a Philosophy of Female Affection*. Beacon Press, Boston; Spinifex Press, North Melbourne.

Raymond, Janice G (1993/1995). *Women as Wombs: Reproductive Technologies and the Battle over Women's Freedom*. Harper Collins, San Francisco; Spinifex Press, North Melbourne.

Raymond, Janice G (2013). *Not a Choice, Not a Job: Exposing the Myths about Prostitution and the Global Sex Trade*. Spinifex Press, North Melbourne.

Responsible Surrogacy (n.d.). 'Information regarding the ethical aspects of the process'; <http://www.r-surrogacy.org/en/>

Ridley, Jane (16 June 2014). 'Child of surrogacy campaigns to outlaw the practice'. *New York Post*; <http://nypost.com/2014/06/16/children-of-surrogacy-campaign-to-outlaw-the-practice/>

Robin, Marie-Monique (2010). *The World According to Monsanto: Pollution, Politics and Power*. Translated by George Holoch, Spinifex Press, North Melbourne.

Rowland, Robyn (1992). *Living Laboratories: Women and Reproductive Technologies.* Pan Macmillan, Sun Books, Sydney; Spinifex Press, North Melbourne; Indiana University Press, Bloomington.

Safi, Michael (14 April 2016). 'Baby Gammy's twin can stay with Australian couple despite father's child sex offences; <https://www.theguardian.com/lifeandstyle/2016/apr/14/baby-gammys-twin-sister-stays-with-western-australian-couple-court-orders>

Sample, Ian (15 December 2016). 'First UK baby with DNA from three people could be born next year'. *The Guardian*; <https://www.theguardian.com/science/2016/dec/15/three-parent-embryos-regulator-gives-green-light-to-uk-clinics>

Sample, Ian (12 January 2017). 'New fertility procedure may lead to "embryo farming," warn researchers'. *The Guardian*; <https://www.theguardian.com/science/2017/jan/11/new-fertility-procedure-may-lead-to-embryo-farming-warn-researchers-in-vitro-gametogenesis>

Sangari, Kumkum (2015). *Solid:Liquid. A (Trans)national Reproductive Formation.* Tulika Books, Delhi.

Saravanan, Sheela (2016). 'Surrogacy and Gender Justice'. *GovernanceNow* pp. 40–42.

Saravanan, Sheela (2018). *Surrogacy Body Bazaar: Transnational Feminism and Reproductive Justice.* Springer Nature Pte. Ltd. Singapore.

Schneider, Jennifer, Jennifer Lahl and Wendy Kramer (2017). 'Long-term breast cancer risk following ovarian stimulation in young egg donors: a call for follow-up, research and informed consent'. *RBM Online*; <http://www.rbmojournal.com/article/S1472-6483(17)30048-2/pdf>

Se Non Ora Quando – Libere (23 March 2017). 'United Nations Resolution against Surrogate Motherhood'; <http://www.stopsurrogacynow.com/wp-content/uploads/2017/04/OnuResolution_-Se-non-ora-quando-Libere-FIRME.pdf>

Selby, Martha (July 2005). 'Narratives of Conception, Gestation, and Labour in Sanskrit Ayurvedic Texts'. *Asian Medicine*, Vol. 1, No. 2, pp. 254–75.

Sibbald, Barbara (29 May 2001). 'Death but one unintended consequence of gene-therapy trial'. *Canadian Medical association Journal* (CMAJ), Vol. 164, No. 11, pp. 1612; <http://www.collectionscanada.gc.ca/eppp-archive/100/201/300/cdn_medical_association/cmaj/vol-164/issue-11/1612.asp>

Singer, Jill (17 March 2009). 'Moralists cry out on Surrogacy'; <http://www.news.com.au/opinion/moralists-cry-out-on-surrogacy/news-story/dae44e9bb686b530158b2a27b57ab04c>

Singer, Peter and Deane Wells (1984). *The Reproduction Revolution: New Ways of Making Babies.* Oxford University, Oxford and Melbourne.

Sloan, Kathy (24 April, 2017). 'Trading on the Female Body: Surrogacy, Exploitation and Collusion by the US Government'; <http://www.thepublicdiscourse.com/2017/04/19109/>

Solis, Raul (25 March 2017). 'Los Vientres de Alquilar: La cara mas brutal del "Gaypitalismo"'. *Paralelo 36 Andalucia;* <https://www.paralelo36andalucia.com/los-vientres-de-alquiler-la-cara-mas-brutal-del-gaypitalismo/>

Son of a Surrogate website. Brian C. (no surname provided, n.d.). 'The Son of a Surrogate'; <http://sonofasurrogate.tripod.com>

Smith, Kyle (3 October 2013). 'Pregnancy Got You Down? No Problem, Outsource Your Babymaking to India.' *Forbes Magazine.*

Spooner, Rania (25 April 2017). 'Science of the Lambs: Researchers perfect artificial womb that works as well as ewe do.' *The Sydney Morning Herald;* <http://www.smh.com.au/national/health/science-of-the-lambs-researchers-perfect-artificial-womb-that-works-as-well-as-ewe-do-20170425-gvrw5v.html>

Stop Surrogacy Now (26 April 2017). 'International Campaign in Spain to call for Abolition of Surrogacy'; <http://www.stopsurrogacynow.com/international-campaigners-in-spain-to-call-for-abolition-of-surrogacy/#sthash.pOPie3D8.DcZ3OtuD.dpbs>.

Sugden, Joanna and Aditi Malhotra (6 November 2015). 'Foreign Couples in Limbo After India Restricts Surrogacy Services'; <https://www.wsj.com/articles/foreign-couples-in-limbo-after-india-restricts-surrogacy-services-1447698601>

Sullivan, Mary (2007). *Making Sex Work: A Failed Experiment with Legalised Prostitution.* Spinifex Press, North Melbourne.

Sutcliffe, AG, CL Williams, ME Jones, AJ Swerdlow, MC Davies, I Jacobs and BJ Botting (September 2015). 'Ovarian tumor risk in women after Assisted Reproductive Therapy (ART); 2.2 million person years of observation in Great Britain'; *Fertility and Sterility,* Vol. 104, Issue 3, e37; <http://www.fertstert.org/article/S0015-0282(15)00614-7/fulltext>

Swedish Government (2016). *Olika vägar till föräldraskap*. Stockholm, English Summary, pp. 47–72; <http://www.regeringen.se/contentassets/e761299bb1a1405380e7e608a47b3656/olika-vagar-till-foraldraskap-sou-201611>

Swiss Info (2015). 'A child is not a commodity, says top Swiss court'; <http://www.swissinfo.ch/eng/surrogate-law_a-child-is-not-a-commodity--says-top-swiss-court/41575816>

Tankard Reist, Melinda (ed) (2006). *Defiant Birth: Women who Resist Medical Eugenics*. Spinifex Press, North Melbourne.

The Center for Bioethics and Culture (2010–2013). 'Eggsploitation'. Documentary directed by Jennifer Lahl. Pleasant Hill, California; <www.eggsploitation.com>

The Center for Bioethics and Culture (2014). 'Breeders: A Subclass of Women?' Documentary directed by Jennifer Lahl. Pleasant Hill, California; <http://breeders.cbc-network.org>

The Center for Bioethics and Culture (2015). 'Eggsploitation: Maggie's Story'. Documentary directed by Jennifer Lahl. Pleasant Hill, California; <http://www.cbc-network.org/maggie/>

The Economist (13 May 2017). Editorial: 'Carrying a child for someone else should be celebrated – and paid'; <http://www.economist.com/news/leaders/21721914-restrictive-rules-are-neither-surrogates-interests-nor-babys-carrying-child>

The Economist (13 May 2017). 'As demand for surrogacy soars, more countries are trying to ban it'; <http://www.economist.com/news/international/21721926-many-feminists-and-religious-leaders-regard-it-exploitation-demand-surrogacy>

The Hague Conference on Private International Law (2016). 'Report of the February 2016 meeting of the experts' group on parentage/surrogacy'; <https://assets.hcch.net/docs/f92c95b5-4364-4461-bb04-2382e3c0d50d.pdf">

The Hague Conference on Private International Law (2017). 'Report of the experts' group on the parentage/surrogacy project (meeting of 31 January – 3 February 2017)'; <https://assets.hcch.net/docs/ed997a8d-bdcb-48eb-9672-6d0535249d0e.pdf>

The Handmaid's Tale (2017). TV series created by Bruce Miller. Based on 1985 novel of the same name by Margaret Atwood. Shown in Australia on SBS. MGM Television in conjunction with White Oak Pictures, USA.

The Telegraph (UK) (2013). 'India bans gay foreign couples from surrogacy'; <http://www.telegraph.co.uk/news/worldnews/asia/india/9811222/India-bans-gay-foreign-couples-from-surrogacy.html>

Tobin, Bernadette (20 April 2015). 'Surrogacy laws may be a bridge too far for Australia'; <http://www.theage.com.au/comment/surrogacy-laws-may-be-a-bridge-too-far-for-australia-20150420-1mosw7.html>

Tyler, Meagan (2016). 'Ten Myths about Prostitution, Trafficking and the Nordic Model' in Caroline Norma and Melinda Tankard Reist (eds.) *Prostitution Narratives: Stories of Survival in the Sex Trade*. Spinifex Press, North Melbourne.

Vines, Gail (3 December 1987). 'Calves a la carte'. *New Scientist*, p. 23.

Vo, Thin and Daniel B Hardy (August 2012). 'Molecular mechanisms underlying the fetal programming of adult diseases'. *Journal of Cell Communication and Signalling*, Vol. 6, No. 3, pp. 139–153. <http://www.ncbi.nlm.nih.gov/pmc/articles/PMC3421023/>

Wade, Matt (17 August 2014). 'Surrogacy, drug trials and commercialising human bodies'. *The Age*; <http://www.theage.com.au/comment/surrogacy-drug-trials-and-commercialising-human-bodies-20140815-104pae.html>

Wadhwa, Vivek (29 July 2017). 'Scientists successfully edit DNA of human embryo for first time'; <http://www.theage.com.au/national/health/scientists-successfully-edit-dna-of-human-embryo-for-first-time-20170728-gxl8dp.html>

Waring, Marilyn (1988). *Counting for Nothing: What Men Value and What Women are Worth*. Bridget Williams Books, Wellington.

Index

Index

If you would like to know more about Spinifex Press,
write to us for a free catalogue, visit our website
or email us for further information.

Spinifex Press
PO Box 105
Mission Beach QLD 4852
Australia

www.spinifexpress.com.au
women@spinifexpress.com.au